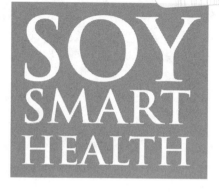

SOY
SMART
HEALTH

SOY
SMART
HEALTH

Discover the "Super Food" that Fights
Breast Cancer, Heart Disease,
Osteoporosis, Menopausal Discomforts,
and Estrogen Dominance

NEIL SOLOMON, M.D., Ph.D.
RICHARD PASSWATER, Ph.D.
RITA ELKINS, M.H.

WOODLAND PUBLISHING
Pleasant Grove, Utah

Note: The information in this book is for educational purposes only and is not recommended as a means of diagnosing or treating an illness. All matters concerning physical and mental health should be supervised by a health practitioner knowledgeable in treating that particular condition. Neither the publisher nor author directly or indirectly dispenses medical advice, nor do they prescribe any remedies or assume any responsibility for those who choose to treat themselves.

Woodland Publishing
P.O. Box 160
Pleasant Grove, Utah
84062
(800) 777-2665
http://www.woodlandpublishing.com

ISBN 1-58054-044-9

Printed in the United States of America.

Contents

Introduction

WHAT IF SOMEONE told you that nature provides compounds called phytoestrogens (plant estrogens) that can help decrease your risk of breast cancer, heart disease and osteoporosis, as well as work to alleviate all kinds of hormonally stimulated problems, including premenstrual and menopausal symptoms? Chances are you'd be a bit skeptical. The truth is that the ordinary soybean more than aptly qualifies as one of these super nutrient-charged foods. Certain compounds contained in soy have the ability to act as both weak estrogens and as estrogen blockers in the human body (no small task). And that's not the whole story. Soy can also prevent cardiovascular problems, prostate diseases and colon cancer, as well as have positive effects on sugar regulation for diabetics. In addition, new studies have found that plant phytoestrogens, like the ones contained in soy, may even be used as a substitute for hormone replacement therapy (HRT) in some women.

It seems that everyone is talking about soy these days. Scientists and medical doctors are gathering together at special symposiums to compare notes on soy, and their findings are impressive. In addition, soy food products, which were found only in "fringe" health food stores ten or fifteen years ago, are now being found in mainstream grocery and other stores. In fact, popular cereal giants Kellogg's and General Mills are currently developing soy breakfast products, and prominent industrial, agricultural, and personal care companies like DuPont, Archer Daniels Midland and Procter & Gamble are also heavily involved in bringing soy food products to our dinner tables.

While soy foods offer all of us significant health benefits, American women in particular need to become acquainted with the profound influence soy has on estrogen pathways. As medical professionals with many years' experience, we have been profoundly concerned with the rising rates of breast, uterine and cervical cancer. Clearly, these diseases are largely the result of hormonal disruptions. Thousands of women in the United States die from breast cancer annually. While we've seen some progress with the application of new drugs and detection methods, the role of diet and phytoestrogenic foods like soy have been grossly neglected. Statistics now report that over half of all cancers in American women have strong links to dietary factors.

Soybeans, which are widely consumed in Asian cultures, have a direct bearing on reducing the risk of certain cancers. In fact, soybeans are a rich source of phytoestrogens that every woman should consider taking advantage of. When it comes to knowledge about soy, ignorance is not bliss, but in a recent survey, over 70 percent of women polled were simply not aware that soy foods could offer them significant protection against breast cancer.

Moreover, scores of women remain confused about HRT, and many believe synthetic hormonal drugs are their only option. However, something as simple as adding soy foods to the diet can play an enormous role in not only lowering the risk of breast cancer but also in elevating the quality of life for so many women who struggle with hormonally-driven symptoms. The epidemic of PMS, menopausal miseries and the serious health implications that these disorders pose for thousands of women are due to what is often called *estrogen dominance*—something that the phytoestrogenic compounds found in soy can help suppress.

While there are various beneficial measures women can take, learning how to use soy effectively should be at the top of any woman's list. In addition, medical doctors should learn more about soy in order to pass reliable information on to their patients. With all the soy hype that's circulating, the likelihood of misinformation is high, bringing to mind Mark Twain's observation that "[t]he trouble with the world is not that people know too little, but that they know so many things that ain't so."

This book, then, is the result of sifting and sorting through mountains of soy data so that you don't have to. It has been written in the hopes that it will enable you to tell the difference between soy fact and fiction. (Keep in mind that soy food manufacturers have now been granted the right by the Food and Drug Administration [FDA] to print certain health advantages on their labels.) Amidst claims that range from the sublime to the ridiculous, one thing remains crystal clear—the Asian diet, which touts more vegetable than animal protein and is low in fat and high in soy foods, has a direct bearing on why Asian women have less breast and endometrial cancers, rarely experience PMS and sail through menopause. Why? Because Asian women have lower circulating estrogen levels than their American sisters do. We are barely beginning to grasp the enormous impact that too much circulating estrogen can have on a woman's reproductive system, not to mention her emotional state. Taking everything into account, the consistent consumption of soy by Asian women emerges as the single most important factor in affording them the hormonal protection that has eluded Western women.

Soy contains plant estrogens that actually work to both block and stimulate estrogen. Its value for American women who struggle with all kinds of estrogen-related maladies cannot be over-emphasized. In a time when synthetic hormones take center stage, using natural estrogens, like the phytoestrogens in soy, to help modulate conditions like PMS and menopause and to prevent the development of breast and endometrial cancers must be addressed. Testing and research also support soy's role in women's health.

Like each of this book's authors, many health professionals recognized long ago that Mother Nature's pharmacopoeia could benefit us all. We have been struck with not only the remarkable health benefits of soy but also the benefits of natural progesterone, omega-3 and omega-9 fatty acids, antioxidant substances, noni, anticancer compounds called indoles that are found in certain vegetables, dietary fiber, a number of botanicals, and the absolute importance of good nutrition to fine tune hormonal balance. Most women fail to appreciate the scope of what natural compounds offer them in terms of viable therapies. Knowledge is the key.

This book discusses why estrogen levels need to be modulated, what soy can and can't do, how to use it wisely with other supplements and dietary changes, and other simple steps that will give women the best natural options available for maximum hormone management. This book is our attempt to take the research data from the health benefits of soy, filter it through over seventy-five collective years of research and clinical experience, and present to you a unique and unbiased point of view about the role soy can play in your life.

chapter 1

Estrogen Can Be Deadly

"It is often the scientist's experience that he senses the nearness of truth when connections are envisioned."

MAHLON HOAGLAND

APPROXIMATELY NINE OF every ten American women endure some type of ailment related to their monthly menstrual cycle, and over half of all women suffer during menopause. Is this what Mother Nature intended? Not likely. For various and little understood reasons, estrogen has taken on an adversarial role in the menstrual cycle of Western women. It is emerging as the primary culprit responsible for so many of the hormonal disturbances we see today. Woman of all ages can become victims of what has been called an estrogen dominance, or estrogen effect, which simply stated, means nothing more than estrogen that is not properly balanced with progesterone.

As concerned health professionals with over seventy-five collective years of research and clinical experience, we ask ourselves why infertility rates have risen and why seemingly healthy young women suffer from menstrual disorders and unprecedented levels of PMS symptoms. In addition, osteoporosis looms as a real threat for thousands of postmenopausal women, and breast cancer kills women of all ages. The fact that so many women plow through their peri- and postmenopausal years perplexed by ills that threaten their emotional and physical well being must also be addressed.

PMS symptoms, such as sore and tender breasts, water retention and emotional swings, affect millions of women. Moreover, the inability to conceive and the incidence of estrogen-stimulated cancers further support the notion that a female hormone imbalance exists for many women.

It is the delicate balance between estrogen and progesterone that drives the menstrual cycle. Interestingly, the total amount of these hormones produced over a woman's lifetime is less than a tablespoon, and yet synchronizing the right ratio of these chemicals profoundly affects not only fertility and conception but overall health as well. Unfortunately, female hormonal equilibrium has been disrupted by a whole host of twentieth-century lifestyle factors, which have impacted circulating levels of estrogen in a majority of women in westernized countries.

This is not to say that estrogen only causes trouble; in fact, this hormone is vital to female development and fertility. In tandem with progesterone (another female hormone made by the ovaries), estrogen regulates the hormonal ups and downs that comprise the 28-day cycle designed to prepare the uterus to receive and nourish a fertilized egg. Estrogen also contributes to the growth of breast tissue and stimulates a number of changes in the female body.

The Positives of Estrogen

While it may seem as though estrogen is mostly a detrimental hormone, certainly all estrogen is not bad. Indeed, estrogen is required for normal female development and reproduction. Estrogen stimulates the changes typically seen in puberty, such as the maturing of the breasts, uterus, fallopian tubes and other parts of the female reproductive system. It is also the hormone that determines how fat will be distributed on the body. One of the reasons that supplemental estrogen is recommended to post-menopausal women is because it also works to protect the heart by boosting high-density lipoproteins (HDLs), or "good" choles-terol, while lowering low-density lipoproteins (LDLs), or "bad" cholesterol. No less important is its ability to prevent bone loss by boosting calcium absorption. Estrogen also helps to keep female skin soft and resilient, and new clinical findings also suggest that estrogen may help to prevent the deterioration of brain cells associated with aging and loss of memory. Estrogen can also impact sexual desire. Clearly, women need estrogen.

What is not commonly understood is that too many pre-menopausal Western women suffer from an estrogen dominance, or estrogen overload, that negatively affects the health and hap-piness of sufferers. The sooner women start their periods and the shorter their cycles are, the longer they will be exposed to the various negative effects of estrogen we just talked about. Vulnerable tissues found in the breast and uterus are estrogen-sensitive, and prolonged exposure to estrogen in these areas can stimulate the growth of cancerous tumors. The first step in pro-tecting yourself from these estrogen risks is learning about how estrogens work. In fact, most women are unaware that there are different types of estrogen and that all estrogens are not created equal.

Estrogen Comes in More than One Form

All estrogens are initially good but can become corrupted through the influence of certain metabolic processes and path-ways. The strongest form of estrogen made in the female body is called 17-beta estradiol. This estrogen needs the most supervision because estradiol, or free estrogen that circulates in the blood-stream, has the ability to stimulate the formation of malignant tumors in breast and endometrial tissue. Fortunately, estradiol can be changed into other forms of estrogen that are not as strong or as potentially dangerous. For example, estriol is another form of estrogen that is made in the placenta and doesn't seem to pose any health risks, and a healthy woman's liver will convert estradiol to estriol on its own. However, estradiol conversion frequently falls short of the body's estriol needs, leaving dangerous estrogen free to circulate through the bloodstream.

The level of available estrogen is regulated by a delicate feedback cycle. Normally, only 1–2 percent of estrogen circulates in the blood, and the remaining amount is bound to protein molecules and is considered inactive or nonthreatening. These estrogen/protein bonds are only broken if the estrogen is needed later by the body. However, because of imbalances in diet and other reasons, many women have above-average levels of free estrogen circulating in their bloodstream.

Estrogen can also play a potentially dangerous role in men as well. Estrogen acts as a precursor compound to male hormones called androgens, which can result in the elevated production of testosterone. Like bad estrogen, bad testosterone has been singled out as the culprit hormone in the development of prostate cancer, which we will discuss in more detail in a later section.

How Does Estrogen Work?

As just described, free estrogens hook up with proteins called estrogen receptors (ERs). These bound molecules, in turn, find a home in special sites located within specific genes in the nucleus of cells. Once inside, these structures can turn the genes on or off—for example, this mechanism makes breast tissue grow during puberty.

For decades, it was thought that only one ER existed, called ER alpha, which targets breast tissue. Since that time, researchers have discovered evidence of another ER, called ER beta. The significance of this ER is its ability to accumulate in other estrogen-sensitive tissues besides breast tissue. While it's obvious that these estrogen processes allow breast development and preserve bone density, they can also prompt the growth of tumors in the breast or bone deterioration if not kept in check.

By the time a woman is postmenopausal, estrogen production declines by almost 70 percent—which is why classic symptoms of "the change" appear. Bones can become more porous and weaker. Hot flashes and night sweats are common, as well as a number of other symptoms discussed in more detail later in this book. However, despite the dramatic decline of estrogen levels, postmenopausal women actually have a higher risk of developing breast cancer. Why is this? The problem has less to do with the total amount of estrogen and more to do with the relationship between estrogen and progesterone and how much of each is circulating in the bloodstream.

Estrogen and progesterone compete for the same receptor sites. In other words, they both want to dock at the same pier. If you have enough circulating progesterone to create a hormonal balance, then less estrogen binds to these sites, and estrogen-driven symptoms and risks decrease. If your progesterone levels are low, however, estrogen takes over and you experience the symptoms of estrogen dominance. This is true even for menopausal women, because progesterone levels also drop during this time, and the resulting drop can create hormonal imbalances as well. The result is still estrogen dominance.

Weight is also a factor. It is thought that the cumulative effects of a lifetime of estrogen exposure and body fat percentage may contribute to a feedback cycle—the more body fat a person carries, the more estrogen she makes. The reverse also holds true—the more estrogen a person make, the easier it is to gain weight and retain fluid.

The Role of Progesterone

Progesterone, also produced in the ovaries, is estrogen's nemesis. Progesterone stimulates the buildup of the uterine lining, which is prepared every month to receive and nourish a fertilized egg. Progesterone also maintains a pregnancy and contributes to the production of breast milk. Mother Nature intended that both estrogen and progesterone offset each other in proper ratios at certain times of the month and during pregnancy. They should work to create a balance that keeps body systems functioning properly for each woman, depending on her age and other factors.

Unfortunately, the hormonal scales of most women are seriously tipped, which disrupts the normal checks and balances that keep estrogen levels from going awry. More often than not, estrogen ends up dominating the menstrual cycles and causes everything from PMS to skipped or heavy periods to dramatic emotional swings. In some cases, menstrual cycles even take place without ovulation (anovulatory cycle), which can also compound the problem of hormonal imbalance. When a premenopausal woman doesn't ovulate, progesterone production is inhibited while estrogen is produced. Consequently, the beneficial opposition normally provided by progesterone is missing, and the problem is compounded the longer it remains out of balance. It's very important to understand too that whether the estrogen is natural or synthetic, if it fails to be opposed by its counterpart, progesterone, an estrogen dominance can result. It's also interesting to note that estrogen dominance seems to be a side effect of industrialized countries and is not commonly seen in "underdeveloped" societies.

How do we know some women aren't ovulating during their cycles? Studies have found that some young women who have regular menstrual cycles did not experience a mid-cycle increase in progesterone levels, suggesting that ovulation did not actually occur. Dr. John Lee, a physician and expert in using natural progesterone, cites this research as yet another example of the widespread incidence of anovulatory cycles occurring in young women throughout the United States—a fact that is undoubtedly linked to rising infertility rates. When these factors are coupled with growing cases of eating disorders, poor nutrition, stress and other factors, hormonal havoc is inescapable, and estrogen is the major contributor.

This imbalanced estrogen environment not only affects women's cancer risks and uterine health but also profoundly impacts how they feel, both physically and emotionally. Many older women assume that because estrogen levels decline with age, their estrogen overload will eventually dissipate. However, it needs to be reiterated that when estrogen output (no matter how small) is unopposed by adequate levels of progesterone, an imbalance occurs, and estrogen will dominate the hormonal landscape.

We have also found that low levels of thyroid hormones, which can occur in cases of hypothyroidism, can also be linked to progesterone deficiencies. In other words, if you lack thyroid hormones, you may be predisposed to an excess of estrogen. Symptoms that point to an underactive thyroid include cold intolerance, weight gain, dry skin, brittle nails, fatigue and irregular periods. Keep in mind that if your doctor finds your hormone levels to be too low, taking excess synthetic thyroid hormones can predispose you to osteoporosis. Taking a good calcium/magnesium supplement with vitamin D (see the chapter on osteoporosis for more detail), as well as an iodine supplement for the thyroid problem, is a good idea.

Are You Estrogen Dominant?

As mentioned earlier, Dr. John Lee, a physician who has done a great deal of investigative work into the role of estrogen dominance, points out that many of the chronic symptoms women typically endure may be due to estrogen dominance. As we also discussed previously, when estrogen is unopposed or unbalanced by progesterone, this estrogen dominance causes undesirable symptoms. Progesterone helps to temper the negative effects of an estrogen surplus. If you suspect that you may suffer from an estrogen dominance, you can ask your doctor to check your hormone levels. Keep in mind, however, that test results may not adequately reflect your true hormonal landscape, which changes from day to day. Personally assessing whether or not you suffer from unopposed estrogen is not difficult; we have found that the following symptoms typically characterize estrogen excess:

- breast enlargement
- breast tenderness
- carbohydrate cravings
- certain types of acne
- cold hands and feet
- depression
- fatigue
- fibrocystic breasts
- fibroid tumors
- headaches
- hypoglycemia
- inability to focus
- inability to maintain a pregnancy
- infertility
- irregular periods
- loss of libido
- mood swings
- PMS
- thyroid dysfunction
- uterine cramping
- water retention
- weight gain (hips and thighs)

Ironically, if you suffer from one or a combination of the above symptoms, your physician may prescribe a synthetic estrogen drug (often a birth control pill) as the treatment of choice. This treatment is more often than not the last thing you need. Because your estrogen levels may be relatively unopposed by progesterone, supplemental synthetic estrogen would only make things worse. In fact, women can be susceptible to an estrogen dominance up to twenty years prior to the onset of menopause, even though hormonal disruptions are typically associated with women in their forties. However, since estrogen dominance can even appear in women in their twenties, this may explain why they often experience severe PMS, mood swings and weight gain. Ask any woman, whether she is twenty or fifty, who battles this phenomenon, and she'll inevitably tell you that weight loss seems almost impossible and that retaining water is as common with her cycle as mood swings. Moreover, an estrogen dominance can also pose serious health risks such as an increased risk for breast or endometrial cancer.

Estrogen dominance can also contribute to the following:

• loss of zinc
• impaired thyroid function
• reduction of cellular oxygenation
• blood sugar disorders
• increased risk of uterine and breast cancer
• increased blood clotting (which raises the risk of stroke)
• increased risk of gallbladder disease (because of thickened bile)

The Estrogen Link to Autoimmune Disease

In addition, recent studies suggest that one of the possible reasons diseases like Lupus afflict many more women than men is the role of fluctuating estrogen levels. In a 1999 study published in *Environmental Health Perspectives,* research scientists reported that in several animal models, estrogens promote B-cell mediated autoimmune diseases. The study supports the notion that estrogen levels can affect and modulate immune responses in the female body.

The research team found that when laboratory animals were given supplemental estrogen, their lymphocyte or white blood cell count decreased. Moreover, the presence of this supplemental estrogen altered the function of T and B cells while stimulating the production of autoantibodies—which can contribute to the development of an autoimmune disease. The study points out that "A striking common feature of many autoimmune diseases in humans and experimental animals, despite differences in pathology, is that females are highly susceptible to autoimmune conditions compared to males." Scientists involved also suggest that xenoestrogens may play a role in the development of autoimmune diseases like lupus.

The researchers continue: "Could environmental estrogens promote some human autoimmune disorders? Is there a link between environmental estrogens and autoimmune disorders, especially since these disorders are reported possibly more frequently? These provocative questions warrant investigation. Our findings on immunomodulatory effects may serve as a benchmark to examine whether endocrine-disrupting chemicals will have similar immunologic effects." This study may also lend some credence to the theory that women can be more susceptible to infections during certain times of their menstrual cycle, especially if they are suffering from an estrogen dominance.

What Causes Estrogen Dominance?

Why do so many women suffer from estrogen excess? No one seems to be adequately addressing this question—certainly this is not what Mother Nature had in mind. The fact is that most North American women typically live a life that drains them both physically and emotionally, while offering them little in terms of replenishment. In other words, in the everyday frenzy of working and raising families in our fast-paced world, good nutrition and health habits are often compromised, while stress levels continue to skyrocket. To make matters worse, environmental pollutants of all kinds surround us daily. Also, the alarming number of young women who suffer from eating disorders is another factor which greatly impacts female reproductive health. Many people also diet regularly, and when they do eat, their food choices often include highly processed foods. We must weigh the health consequences of eating fragmented, chemically altered and unnaturally preserved foods.

With the addition of aspartame and olestra to our snack repertoire, we are now eating non-food substitutes as if they were the real things. Similarly, many fresh vegetables and fruits no longer contain the mineral content they once did due to stripped soils. The mineral content of that fresh broccoli or orange you're eating depends on the mineral content of the soil in which it grows.

If the soil is depleted of minerals, so is its harvest. A deficiency of even just one mineral can impair hormonal balance, as well as thousands of other biochemical reactions in the body. Moreover, hidden environmental hormones found in plant sources can originate from pesticides. Other chemicals also have an impact on our reproductive hormones.

chapter 2

Today's Endocrine Disruptors

"The human body has been designed to resist an infinite number of changes and attacks brought about by its environment. The secret of good health lies in successful adjustment to changing stresses on the body."

HARRY J. JOHNSON

THE ENDOCRINE SYSTEM, comprised of various glands, produces a variety of hormones that control our growth and reproduction. Some of the major endocrine glands include the pituitary, thyroid, parathyroid, pancreas, adrenal and the male and female gonads (testes and ovaries). Endocrine glands make and secrete hormones directly into the bloodstream. Hormones are remarkable chemical messengers that come in contact with tissues, organs and cells throughout the body by binding to specific cell sites called receptors. This lock and key effect triggers various responses in affected tissues. However, external chemicals, called endocrine disruptors, have the ability to interfere with or manipulate these essential hormonal pathways and change hormonal responses in our bodies.

Laboratory studies tell us that these substances can impact virtually any mechanism of the endocrine system—from hormone production to receptor site binding and the normal breakdown of circulating hormones. In fact, many chemicals, including certain pesticides, can damage the workings of the endocrine system and can cause everything from ovarian dysfunction to impaired sperm production. These damages to the workings of the endocrine system then cause a destructive chain reaction that affects our overall health.

Environmental Estrogens

Environmental estrogens are considered both natural and synthetic chemicals capable of interfering with the function of both estrogen and testosterone. Some environmental estrogens impact the estrogen binding sites found in breast, prostate and other tissue, while others just mimic estrogen itself and can have a wide variety of effects, such as the inhibition of male hormones or the stimulation of estrogen-related symptoms. This chapter covers environmental estrogens with negative effects, like certain pesticides, the pill and other synthetics, as well as natural environmental estrogens with positive effects, like phytoestrogens (including the soybean). Also, we will discuss how issues like diet, stress and the mineral content of soils affect hormone balance.

The Impact of Xenoestrogens

Xenoestrogens refer to a group of synthetic chemicals with estrogenic actions. Most of these xenoestrogens are resistant to degradation, so they can inhabit the body for long periods of time. Xenoestrogens of this type include organic pollutants such as polychlorinated biphenyls, chlorinated pesticides, DDT, plasticizers in PVC pipe, bisphenol (found in food can coatings), polycarbonate plastics (PCBs), resins used in dentistry, alkylphenol ethoxylates (found in many detergents) and dioxins released from industrial plants into water supplies. Even the plastic wrap seals we see on virtually everything at our corner market may contain endocrine disruptors, which can mimic or block hormones in the body. A plasticizer agent used in some plastic wraps may contain a chemical called di-(2-ethylhexyl) adipate, or DEHA, which gives these wraps their ability to cling. This chemical is considered a threat to the endocrine system. Research has shown that it can leach into food that it touches, especially if that food has a high fat content.

The Consumer's Union conducted a test with nineteen pieces of prewrapped cheese and found that seven of the samples wrapped in the PVC plastics contained alarmingly high levels of DEHA. While more studies are needed to assess the dangers of eating foods wrapped with PVC plastic products, the fact remains that unseen endocrine disruptors are present in our everyday, seemingly safe environments. We can protect ourselves by repackaging our foods, cutting off the outer edges of foods like cheeses or meats before we eat them, and by using paper wraps before we store food items in a plastic bag. We should also never heat up food covered with plastic in the microwave. In addition, the Environmental Protection Agency (EPA) is in the process of screening scores of chemicals to assess whether or not they interfere with endocrine functions in the human body.

The DES Disaster

The devastating effect of diethylstilbestrol (DES), one of the first synthetic, nonsteroidal estrogen drugs, is well documented and is a sad commentary on the hidden dangers of prescription drugs. This chemical increased the risk of vaginal and cervical cancers in women who were exposed to the drug as fetuses. Somewhere between four and six million American and European women and 10,000 Australian women used DES for the prevention of miscarriage and pregnancy complications. The drug was prescribed for a variety of other conditions ranging from acne to prostate cancer. It took decades before scientists discovered that DES was dangerous. Reports surfaced that twenty years after taking DES, women had a 40–50 percent greater risk of breast cancer than nonexposed women did. Moreover, children born to these women showed an abnormally high incidence of reproductive abnormalities, miscarriages, vaginal cancer, testicular cancer, sterility and immune dysfunction. Assessing the ultimate levels of damage DES has caused and will continue to cause is virtually impossible.

For instance, from 1977 to 1979, an epidemic of breast enlargement in children was seen in Italy. This epidemic was eventually blamed on DES ingestion from meat sources. Meats and dairy products contain unseen hormones that inevitably impact our reproductive systems. The phenomenon of premature puberty may be related to the fact that our children are often receiving estrogen in their hot dog or drumstick. However, to date, no one has thoroughly addressed the potential risks of hormonally fattened beef, pork and poultry.

Oral Contraceptives and Suppressed Ovulation: Is There a Price Tag?

And lastly, the impact of oral contraceptives must also be considered. The safety of oral contraceptives is a controversial issue because the use of birth control pills is still considered a risk factor for breast cancer, cardiovascular disease and liver and cervical cancers.

Birth control pills made their debut in 1960, and nothing has been the same since. These pills made effective contraception possible in an extremely easy and hassle free way. Since its introduction, "the pill" has been used by more than sixty million women worldwide. It is estimated that approximately five million women in this country used birth control pills in 1973, and

THE IMPACT OF ESTROGEN IMPOSTERS

The impact of estrogen imposters on the human body can be tremendous. Our experience, as well as that of other doctors and researchers, clearly indicates that pseudoestrogens can cause a whole host of problems, including:

- Reduction of sperm count and quality
- Increased incidence of male genital abnormalities
- Increased incidence of testicular, prostate and breast cancers
- Increased occurrence of endometriosis
- Premature puberty

records put that figure at over ten million. The pill is by far the most popular birth control method, excluding surgical procedures. However, what we have actually witnessed over the last few decades is enormous numbers of women taking a synthetic hormonal drug for extended periods of time. We can only begin to guess what the long-term health implications are when healthy women ingest synthetic hormones for many years.

The original birth control pill was high in both estrogen and progestin (a synthetic form of progesterone), but by the mid 1970s, oral contraceptives contained 50 micrograms or less of estrogen, which was a significant drop from the 150 micrograms typically taken during the sixties. Progestin amounts also dropped from 10 milligrams to between 2.5 milligrams and 0.15 milligrams. Shortly after this, the FDA approved low-dose pills that contained 20 to 35 micrograms of estrogen. Most pills prescribed today contain 30 to 35 micrograms of estrogen and 0.5 to 1.0 milligram of progestin—a marked improvement. Also, triphasic pills are available that actually change the ratio of progestin to estrogen during the 21-day cycle.

Despite the marked improvement in birth control pills, scores of women took these pills at the higher doses for many years. The effects of this trend are still not completely known, but the FDA is definitely concerned—concerned enough that in 1988, it strongly urged the withdrawal from the market of any pill with over 50 micrograms of estrogen.

How Does the Pill Work?

The pill supplies the body with an oral dose of both estrogen and progestin in much higher than normal levels. By so doing, stimulation of the pituitary gland to produce hormones that would normally prompt ovulation is blocked, but it's not the only organ affected. Virtually every system comes in contact with these potent synthetic hormones. Continually suppressing ovulation may be one reason why there are so many abnormalities in the menstrual cycle today. By having periods and not ovulating, women are at a greater risk for estrogen dominance due to suppressed progesterone production. This estrogen overload can cause the abnormal buildup of the uterine lining because it may not be sufficiently shed. The incomplete removal of the endometrium may lead to endometriosis, uterine fibroid cysts, fibrocystic breasts, bloating, depression, heavy or irregular periods and possible malignancies.

The Safety of Progestins

When it comes to the safety and long term effects of oral contraception, the truth is that medical science continues to supply us with conflicting data. Even the progestin addition to birth control pills and HRT combinations has sparked controversy. Remember that a progestin is a synthetic version of progesterone. What must be stressed here is that even progestins have been linked to the development of breast cancer.

One study conducted at the Department of Human Oncology at the University of Wisconsin Comprehensive Cancer Center in Madison looked at the estrogenic action of progestins and concluded, "A rigorous evaluation of the 'total' estrogenic potential of OC [oral contraceptives] might produce a better correlation with breast cancer risk." Another study designed by Italian scientists addressed all the conflicting data surrounding progestins and stated, "Epidemiological studies have provided conflicting results, ranging from a protective effect to a deleterious effect of progestin addition on breast cancer risk. Progestins include a large family of molecules characterised by different binding capacities to androgen receptors. This implies that they should be considered as distinct yet related therapeutic agents."

Researchers at the University of Colorado caution, "Our data and that of others are beginning to show that one cannot approach the question of progestin actions in isolation. Other important regulatory proteins, whose expression may vary in tissue-specific ways, work in concert with progesterone to decide cell fate. The timing and dose of progesterone may also influence the biological response. Since progestins are widely used in oral contraception, in hormone replacement therapy, and in cancer treatments, it is becoming critically important that the subtleties of their mechanisms of action be clearly understood."

Concerning the use of progestins and breast cancer, a study published in a 1995 issue of the *New England Journal of Medicine* reported: "The addition of progestins to estrogen therapy does not reduce the risk of breast cancer among postmenopausal women. The substantial increase in the risk of breast cancer among older women who take hormones suggests that the trade-offs between risks and benefits should be carefully assessed."

To reiterate, we simply don't know how progestins will affect hormonally sensitive tissue in the long run. Our discussion on birth control pills and their potential risk is based on current information available and is founded on the notion that synthetic hormones are nothing to play around with. The primary question still remains: over the long run, how do oral contraceptives affect a woman's natural estrogen/progesterone relationship? We just don't know.

Other Side Effects Associated with Oral Contraceptives

While the possible cardiovascular side effects of birth control pills (including blood clots, stroke and heart attack) continue to stir controversy on both sides of the fence, the pill's link to cancer is still unclear. Although the pill is purported to lower the risk of ovarian and endometrial cancer, it may stimulate breast cancer. After all, birth control pills are nothing more than synthetic forms of natural hormones, and whenever we take a compound from nature and artificially synthesize it, unwanted side effects may occur.

Does the pill cause cancer or not? An FDA advisory committee has decided that more time and additional research is needed to adequately assess this link. If you are one of thousands of women who take birth control pills every day, this conclusion leaves you in a precarious place. And though your doctor may tell you not to worry, the possibility that the pill causes breast or cervical cancer in some women has not been ruled out. In fact, there are currently no cancer studies available on low-dose birth control pills.

Other potential side effects of the pill include weight gain, mood swings, circulatory and vascular problems and gastrointestinal upset. Blood clots and possible liver problems are also considered real risks. What is ultimately the most troubling issue surrounding birth control side effects is that the majority of women who use oral contraceptives are on the younger side, which poses unanswered questions about their future health. We believe one of the most troubling long-term aspects of the pill is its impact on nutrition.

The Pill's Nutritional Impact

We know now that the pill can create nutritional deficiencies and imbalances and that if you take it, you need to boost your nutritional intake. For example, the need for B-vitamins, particularly pyridoxine (B6) and folic acid, is greater when birth control pills are taken. Vitamin B6 plays a profound role in the production of a neurochemical in the brain called serotonin, which regulates mood, hunger and sleep. Low levels of this vitamin in the body have been linked to depression and other emotional disorders. In addition, folic acid breaks down a compound called homocysteine. High levels of homocysteine have been associated with an increased risk for osteoporosis in postmenopausal women. An article published in the 1960s by the *American Journal of Clinical Nutrition* stated that women on oral contraceptives are more susceptible to osteoporosis in later years because of diminished levels of magnesium. The pill affects the level of magnesium that is absorbed by the body because of its effect on homocysteine levels.

Another link between the pill and depression is the fact that women who take the pill have higher copper levels and lower levels of zinc. This change has been linked to emotional instability. Clearly, many women have pronounced mood swings while taking the pill. This reaction isn't so surprising—if natural hormones can have a big effect on behavior, imagine what havoc strong artificial hormones could cause. In addition, if ovulation is suppressed, natural estradiol and progesterone levels decline, which also impacts mood.

There is also some speculation that the need for vitamins C, E and K may be increased when taking birth control pills. In addition, using birth control pills may also cause an alkaline imbalance in the vaginal canal, which could lead to increased infection. Simply stated, synthetic hormones have a dark side; women must decide if the pros of the pill outweigh the cons. Clearly, the pill has impacted the delicate balance of female hormones in both positive and negative ways.

Typical American Eating Habits and Their Hormonal Implications

Assessing the health impacts of the American diet on the average person could fill volumes. However, zeroing in on how the typical Western diet has affected the reproductive and endocrine system of women is difficult, to say the least. Our edibles just aren't what they used to be. We now routinely consume new

MALNUTRITION AMIDST PLENTY

It has been estimated that less than 10 percent of Americans eat a balanced diet. Here are more frightening statistics:

- Only one in nine people eats the recommended number of servings of fruits and vegetables.

- The average level of calcium consumption in the United States and Canada is two-thirds of the RDA of 800 milligrams.

- Americans are eating increasingly more sugar and refined grains that are depleted of vitamins and minerals.

- Fifty-nine percent of Americans' calories come from potentially nutrient-poor food sources (e.g., soft drinks, white bread and snack foods). These poor food choices result in sub-optimal levels of essential vitamins and minerals being consumed.

- Many diets in the United States provide only half the recommended amounts of folic acid.

- Only one person in five consumes adequate levels of vitamin B6.

- Nine out of ten diets require marginal levels of chromium, as well as vitamin A, C, B1, B2, B6, iron, copper and zinc.

- As many as 20 percent of people hospitalized for depression lack vitamin B6.

- Women in particular are at risk nutritionally because they continually restrict calories, lose iron through their periods and frequently take birth control pills, which can lower certain nutrient levels.

crops that have been genetically engineered. Our beef, poultry and pork are commonly injected with hormones for quick fattening. High-tech processing techniques and chemical preservatives inhibit the natural deterioration of processed meats like sausage or salami.

Unlike our grandparents, we no longer eat foods in season. Fruits and vegetables are shipped transcontinentally and are often packed in dry ice or in cold storage for extended periods of time. Moreover, new foods and synthetic food substitutes like aspartame and newly emerging "fake fats" like olestra are rapidly dominating our selection of grocery store foods. Olestra, for example, can interfere with the absorption of fat-soluble vitamins like E, A, K and D. Consequently, supplementation of these vitamins is required to offset this effect.

Ironically, some of our foods act more like "antifoods" in that they serve to inhibit or destroy nutrients rather than to supply them. For example, the phosphorus content found in many soft drinks causes the body to leech out calcium, and sugar coupled with caffeine deplete the body of B vitamins and other essential nutrients.

Soil Depletion

In a past issue of *August Celebration*, Linda Grover made a very enlightening and somewhat alarming statement. She said that in 1948 spinach had 158 milligrams of iron, but by 1965, the maximum amount of iron in spinach had dropped to 27 milligrams. In 1973, it was averaging 2.2 milligrams—that's down from 158 milligrams. Today you would have to eat seventy-five bowls of spinach to get the same amount of iron that one bowl could have given you back in 1948. She reminds us that Popeye was very popular about that same time, and now we know one reason why this might be. Spinach is just not what it used to be. Interestingly, women who suffer from heavy periods are prone to become iron deficient or anemic, and eating fresh spinach is not going to resupply iron stores the way it once could have.

Scientists have determined that at least twenty-six minerals are "bottom line" critical for balanced nutrition. Even if we lack a few vitamins, the body can still make some use of minerals, but when we lack minerals, vitamins are useless. The alarming fact is that even if you are eating a well-balanced diet, you're probably among the 95 percent of Americans who are lacking in at least one major mineral! Mineral-poor soil is a major causal factor. As far back as 1936, U.S. Senate Document No. 264 warned Americans that the soils used to grow fruits and vegetables were seriously deficient in minerals. Continuous cropping and pollution were robbing our soil of the minerals needed to sustain life, and today the situation has not improved. Another disturbing government report from the 1992 Earth Summit shows that our earth's soil is anemic. In North America, 85 percent of the minerals in farm and range soils have been depleted over the last 100 years. How does this mineral depletion affect hormonal balances? We can only surmise at this point that it is one of many contributing factors to the high incidence of Western diseases and health problems that we see today.

High Sugar and Fat Consumption

Jeff Arder once said, "We live in an age when pizza gets to your home before the police!" We Americans love our fast food, and it is full of calories, fats and sugar. In the *Journal of Reproductive Medicine*, a 1991 article stated that the consumption of food and drink high in sugar is linked to the prevalence of PMS. The average American eats over 125 pounds of white sugar every year. It has been estimated that sugar makes up 25 percent of our daily calorie intake, with soda pop supplying the majority of that intake. Americans eat an average of fifteen quarts of ice cream per person per year.

These numbers are even more shocking considering that sugar, in excess amounts, can be toxic. Sufficient amounts of B vitamins are required to even metabolize and detoxify the sugar in our bodies. A high sugar diet and lack of B vitamins have been linked to depression. Interestingly, because birth control pills also inhibit the utilization of B vitamins, women who eat high sugar diets have a greater risk of becoming depressed.

Sugar and Serotonin

The Wurtman study published in *Scientific American* made a compelling correlation between brain serotonin levels and constant carbohydrate cravings. This study indicated that when brain levels of serotonin decreased in the test subjects, some people started to crave carbohydrates. This same serotonin factor has been linked to PMS symptoms as well, especially cravings and irritability, because research indicates that estrogen levels can affect serotonin amounts in the brain. The study also points out that in some people who have trouble with mood swings or PMS, the brain fails to respond as it should when starchy snacks are eaten. Therefore, the craving persists and overeating occurs.

Fiber and Fat

In short, America is the most overfed and undernourished society in the world. Eating diets high in polyunsaturated, hydrogenated and saturated fats and low in fiber has also dealt a profound blow to our overall health. And since breast cells store fat, if women eat dangerous fats, these fats will inevitably end up in the breast tissue. Moreover, a 1996 study conducted at the Oncology Department of St. Thomas Hospital in London concluded that case-control studies in various populations around the world have reported a lower risk of breast cancer as linked with a higher intake of dietary fiber and complex carbohydrates. The study reported, "Although this finding has not been confirmed through American studies, the scope of its observations strongly support the notion that increasing the consumption of fiber or the use of dietary fiber supplements might reduce breast cancer risk in high-incidence populations." Fiber, in fact, works in a number of ways to prevent estrogen-stimulated cancers.

Estrogen and Elimination

Constipation has become so prevalent in this country that most of us hardly acknowledge it as a legitimate medical condition. Women are especially prone to sluggish bowel and can easily become laxative dependent. Poor bowel elimination also poses additional threats to women, since significant amounts of estrogen are excreted in bowel movements. If a woman has dangerous estradiol levels, then the problem is compounded if her body can't eliminate excess estrogen. These estrogens, which find their way into the intestines from the liver as a constituent of bile, must be properly eliminated. When estrogen-laced waste sits in the bowel for twenty-four hours or more, estrogen can be reabsorbed back into the body. In fact, a Tuft's University study found that lower blood estrogen levels correlated with heavier stool weight, suggesting that estrogen is continually eliminated through bowel movements. (By the way, to illustrate that hormones are indeed excreted in waste material, the widespread use of birth control pills and HRT have actually resulted in the synthetic estrogen pollution of many of our lakes and rivers by way of our sewage systems.)

Estrogen and Salt

Women often crave salty snacks or over-salt their food. It is now thought that estrogen may be affected by salt intake. To make matters worse, if estrogen dominates, it contributes to a type of sodium potentiation that causes water to attach to its molecules, which further aggravates fluid retention. When cell water pressure rises in the nervous system, headaches and feelings of agitation may occur. Bloating, which is a common symptom of PMS, also causes weight gain. Excess salt intake, another rather common attribute of the American diet, heightens other hormonally driven symptoms.

The Role of Stress

No one really appreciates the profound role that stress can play in determining our physical health. Some experts believe that up to 90 percent of all physical illnesses are related to stress. From experience, we can tell you that stress directly impacts the release of certain hormones that intrinsically influence virtually every major body system. For example, when you feel stressed, brain chemicals are altered and messages are sent to your adrenal glands, which prompts the release of adrenal hormones including those that excite the nervous system and impact the ratios of other hormones like estrogen and progesterone. Adrenal output also includes the release of cortisosteroids, which enter our circulatory systems and predispose us to the "fight or flight" phenomenon, which can put undo strain on our immune responses. Consequently, our body may become more vulnerable to neoplastic (cancer-causing) and damaging heart and blood pressure processes in the presence of these chemicals, which are capable of accelerating cancer-causing and heart disease cascades. Hormones made in the adrenal and pituitary glands, which include cortisol, adrenaline and prolactin, inhibit the activities of white blood cells, decrease the amount of lymphocytes produced and may cause the thymus gland to actually shrink.

Stress and Cancer: Is There a Link?

Stress must be recognized as a probable causal factor for cancer. In fact, studies have found that the incidence of breast cancer was significantly higher in the women who had experienced a traumatic emotional experience during the six years before they developed the tumor. Many other studies support the very damaging effects of stress on immunity, pointing out that T-cell activity is dramatically impaired in people who lose their spouses, lose their jobs or experience other emotionally upsetting events. When the stress becomes severe enough and chronic in nature, chemical changes occur in the body that inadvertently create an environment which may predispose us to disease.

Women who carry extra-heavy stress loads need to realize that unless they lower their stress levels or learn to manage them better, their hormonal health is in peril. According to a report published in *Neuroscience and Biobehavioral Review* in 1992, estrogens may actually be released from the adrenal glands and the ovaries during periods of psychological stress, predisposing a woman to an excess of estrogen.

A *Simple Stress Test*

Scientists have certain criteria for evaluating individual stress levels to determine whether or not stress is reaching the kind of level that needs additional management. We have used this test in our research and found that it correlates well to individuals who have stress-prone personalities. If you answer yes to two or more of the following questions, you probably have a stress-prone personality:

- Do you try to do more than one thing at a time?
- Do you rush through your meals?
- Are you compulsive about punctuality?
- Do you find it difficult to relax?
- Do others tell you to take things slower?
- Do you interrupt others frequently while they are talking?
- Are you accident-prone?
- Do you get impatient or upset if something or someone delays you (such as traffic jams, appointments, etc.)?

Doctors often treat the symptoms of stress with tranquilizers and antidepressant drugs. Using barbiturate hypnotic drugs or narcotic analgesics, however, is not the ideal way to manage anxiety or even insomnia. The tendency to prescribe drugs for stress is characteristic of the attitude of some physicians who feel compelled to come up with quick pharmaceutical fixes for women's problems, when lifestyle, diet and emotional problems are what really need attention.

Keep in mind that stress alone is bad enough, but when you couple stress with malnutrition, pollution, spiritual disillusionment and other factors, you create a situation that can profoundly disrupt your delicate hormonal relationships and affect your overall mental and physical health.

Summary of Conditions Linked to an Estrogen/Progesterone Imbalance

To put it simply, when estrogen is inadequately opposed by progesterone for whatever reason, the fragile balance of female health can be jeopardized. If you suffer from estrogen-related maladies, then any one of the following factors may predispose you to this imbalanced hormonal scenario:

- malnutrition and stress
- taking synthetic estrogens (HRT, birth control pills, etc.)
- lack of ovulation (commonly seen in perimenopause—the years prior to menopause—but can be seen in younger women)
- exposure to xenoestrogens or estrogen-like compounds found in the environment and food supply
- hysterectomies

Studies have also shown that potentially dangerous forms of estrogen-mutants and toxic forms of estradiol and estrone have been linked to the following factors:

- high-fat diets
- excessive alcohol intake
- obesity
- low thyroid function
- exposure to pesticide residues

So what can be done to counteract the negative effects of all these endocrine disruptors? Using certain compounds from nature, such as phytoestrogens, can offer us (especially women) significant health benefits.

Phytoestrogens to the Rescue

An ancient Chinese proverb says that a time of crisis can also be a time of great opportunity. In the midst of widespread hormonal disruption, we have the chance to utilize plants that can literally work wonders to help restore hormonal balance. Unquestionably, our bodies were originally designed to consume plants, not just to sustain life but also to protect us from potentially dangerous health threats. Scientists are just beginning to appreciate the impressive array of nutrients and non-nutrients found in plants that drive our body systems and help neutralize harmful chemical invaders.

Phyto is Greek for plant and is used to prefix nutrients, estrogens, etc. Phytoestrogens describe certain compounds found in plants that have the ability to act as weak estrogens or other sex hormones in the human body. Unlike synthetic estrogens, phytoestrogens exert positive effects on the human body. Why are there hormonal compounds in plants? Some scientists believe plants make phytoestrogens to defend themselves from plant-eating predators, much in the same way that plants make thorns or thistles. Animals that continually eat phytoestrogenic plants may become fertility impaired. Decreasing these animal populations increases the plant's chances for survival, because fewer animals mean less plant consumption. These powerful phytochemicals were designed to exert a specific effect on mammals and insects that pose a natural threat to plants. Phytochemicals also protect these plants from oxidative damage, a benefit that carries over to our own human body systems.

Phytoestrogens have now been identified in some 300 plants and are grouped in the following categories:

- coumestans (bean sprouts, red clover and sunflower seeds)
- lignans (rye, wheat, sesame seeds and linseed)
- isoflavones (some fruits and vegetables, but primarily soybeans and soy products)

Beets, rye grass, wheat, alfalfa, clover, apples and cherries all have a weak estrogenic action. A few of the other herbs and berries that have recently been recognized for their phytoestrogenic properties include the following:

- chaste berry (also known as vitex), an herb thought to increase progesterone production and balance estrogen and progesterone.
- black cohosh root, which was traditionally used by Native Americans for menstrual cramps.
- dong quai, an herb prescribed throughout Asia for various female problems, including hot flashes.

The Natural Estrogenic Effect of Phytoestrogens

Unlike synthetic hormone drugs, plants with estrogenlike substances appear to naturally support the female reproductive system. These substances make the plants useful for a number of disorders including breast, endometrial and prostate cancer prevention; menopausal and PMS miseries; and osteoporosis prevention. Phytoestrogens have the unique ability to compete with human estrogens for tissue receptor sites. In basic terms, this means that the plant estrogens attach to the tissues where human estrogens normally would. Therefore, less human estrogen is able to attach to receptors. By introducing phytoestrogens to the body, we are able to decrease the activity of dangerous estrogens (like estradiol) while promoting a healthy balance of estrogen to progesterone in the body. Phytoestrogens also inhibit certain enzymatic reaction involved in the growth of cancerous cells and boost body mechanisms that help to keep estrogen levels in check. These plants also contain an impressive array of other phytonutrients that provide powerful cellular protection, especially against cancer.

Phytoestrogen Levels and Cancer

A fascinating study, which illustrates just how important the relationship of phytoestrogens to cancer really is, involves a case-controlled study published in a 1997 edition of *Lancet*. The study was designed to evaluate the link between phytoestrogen consumption and the risk of breast cancer. Women who had newly-diagnosed and early stages of breast cancer were interviewed, and a blood sample and 72-hour urine collection were taken before any treatment started. After considering factors such as age at menopause, alcohol and total fat intake, researchers concluded that it was the high levels of phytoestrogens in the urine that were associated with substantially lower breast-cancer risks. In other words, the more phytoestrogens consumed and the higher the level of phytoestrogens in urine, the less risk for cancer.

Research data like this tells us that because phytoestrogens can be detected in human urine and blood samples, these compounds are absorbed after ingestion and enter the bloodstream. In addition, they can be converted into other compounds considered estrogenic. In contrast to the dangerous synthetic estrogens we discussed, phytoestrogens are easily broken down and are not stored in human tissue. In other words, they spend a relatively short amount of time in the body before they are metabolized and excreted.

In fact, it is expedient that the American public become informed about the need to incorporate certain foods containing phytonutrients into their diets in order to prevent diseases like cancer. Simple dietary changes—now backed by scientific data—are infinitely safer than turning to pharmaceutical agents. The complex synergy of each compound in a plant proves that no isolated or artificially synthesized drug can equal the effect of a whole food.

The Superiority of Whole Phytoestrogenic Foods

Phytoestrogenic plants have been intrinsically designed with a wide array of inherent components that complement each other and work more efficiently when they are kept together. Like isolating pharmaceutical agents from herbs to create synthetic drugs (which have various bad side effects), separating the phytoestrogenic constituents from these plants may not be desirable. In her book *Foods and Healing*, author Annmarie Colbin writes:

> [I]nstead of eating a vegetable in the shape in which it grows, we consume it in fragmented form, its separate components split apart, we are not following the natural scheme of things. When we consume wheat germ, white flour and bran separately, it is not the same as eating them in their natural, integrated and properly balanced state as whole wheat. . . . A hundred or so years ago, it was discovered that stripping the bran and germ off the wheat made the flour not only whiter and fluffier, but also longer-lasting. . .soon I was eating white bread and putting wheat germ in the meat loaf. Isn't this the ultimate irony? We take what is originally a perfect food, fragment it and refine it, and then we purchase its separated components individually to add back to other foods.

Current data, which is slowly emerging, strongly suggests that we look at the value of whole plant foods very carefully. When cereal grains, fruits, vegetables, beans, nuts and seeds are tampered with, altered or fragmented, they become artificial foods to some extent. The notion of "wholesomeness" cannot be dismissed. It is intrinsically valuable in nature's food storehouse, especially when it comes to phytoestrogens.

Are Phytoestrogens Safe?

Because phytoestrogens have turned the scientific community on their ear, possible risks associated with using them need to be addressed. First of all, eating very high levels of some phytoestrogenic plants may pose some health risks. For example, in one study animals that ate diets comprised of almost 100 percent phytoestrogen-rich plants experienced reproductive impairment. Another concern centers on the effects of phytoestrogens on infants or children. For example, some phytoestrogens may interfere with the endocrine development in a baby while protecting adults against breast and prostate cancer (refer to a later section on soy formulas for infants).

However, test studies have found that humans actually have built-in mechanisms to protect themselves from continuous exposure to phytoestrogens but not to synthetic environmental estrogens called xenoestrogens. These studies concluded that large amounts of phytoestrogens like isoflavones can be consumed daily by humans, especially in a vegetarian diet. Many phytoestrogens, such as lignans and isoflavonoids, are metabolized and excreted in urine much like endogenous estrogens produced in the body; therefore, phytoestrogens may not bio-accumulate in the body.

Common-Sense Use of Phytoestrogens

Common sense should, of course, rule when deciding to incorporate phytoestrogens into the diet. Eating raw soybeans or overdosing on phytoestrogenic compounds is obviously not recommended. Keep in mind, however, that you do have to consume large amounts of these plant foods to cause fertility concerns. Using these supplements wisely and in combination with a variety of foods is the key to avoiding any potential adverse effects. Remember also that herbs must be properly used—too much or too little of certain phytoestrogens can be a problem.

In a later section, we'll define what dietary levels of soy are considered safe at this point in time, but clearly there is much we still need to learn about phytoestrogens. What we do know is that consuming these types of plants helps to regulate the kind of hormonal disruption already talked about, according to research. And the fact that these marvelous compounds do exist in nature supports why we were designed to eat plants—something many of us have strayed from. Soybeans and soy-based foods such as tofu contain some of the most beneficial phytoestrogens available. That's why using soy for optimal hormonal balance and protection is the main focus of this book.

chapter 3

The Soybean: Phytoestrogen Extraordinaire

"The man who questions opinions is wise. The man who quarrels with facts is a fool."
ANONYMOUS

FIFTEEN YEARS AGO, very few of us paid attention to what we considered a rather boring legume called the soybean. Now, large-scale symposiums attended by scores of doctors and scientists are held to discuss the extraordinary properties of soy. Almost overnight, the soybean has emerged as one of the earth's "super-foods," because it is low in saturated fat, cholesterol-free, protein-rich and user-friendly.

And now, soy foods are found not only in local health-food stores, but they are also on the shelves of some of the largest grocery chains in the country, featuring brands from companies like breakfast cereal manufacturer Kellogg's.

Unlike other beans, the soybean is composed of 36 percent protein, containing an impressive mix of amino acids, saponins (plant compounds that can lower cholesterol, among other things), phytic acid, trypsin inhibitors, fiber and isoflavones. These soy biochemicals work together to create one food heavy-weight. The saponins and trypsin inhibitors found in soy bind to bile acids and inhibit them from stimulating tumor formation or growth. The fiber content of soy also helps to regulate fat absorption, and soy's phytic acid works to chelate minerals like iron and calcium in the digestive system for better assimilation. In addition, soy possesses something called a Bowman-Birk Inhibitor (BBI), a protease inhibitor that suppresses the growth of both benign and malignant tumors in the liver, lung and colon.

However, it is the phytoestrogenic power of the soybean that we are most concerned with. Ironically, while the merits of soy for women has gained impressive scientific support, most women remain relatively unaware that increasing their soy consumption could be one of the smartest health moves they make.

Asian Women vs. American Women

Soy became marked for vigorous investigation after statistics surfaced which confirmed that Asian women have significantly lower incidences of estrogen-related diseases and disorders such as breast cancer, PMS and menopausal symptoms. Asian women have breast cancer rates often up to ten times lower than American women. Chinese women, who eat an average of fifty grams of soy daily, lower their risk of breast cancer by more than 50 percent. Japanese women consume 50 to 80 grams of soy each day (two to three ounces) and tend to be much less prone to PMS. In addition, they don't even have an equivalent word for "hot flashes" in their vocabulary. By comparison, American women struggle with menopause and spend most of their post-adolescent life coping with hormonally linked ailments. This profound difference in experience further supports research that soy and perhaps other elements in Asian diets promote women's health far better than the current American diet.

Since ancient times, the Asian diet has been rich in soy foods. When looking at the overall health of the Japanese people, we cannot ignore certain statistics. Overall, Japanese people have lower rates of colon, breast, prostate and lung cancer than Americans do. They also live longer—due, in part, to the fact that they have one of the lowest rates of cardiovascular disease for both men and women. And while other factors such as the fiber or vegetable content of their diet must also play a role, their soybean consumption in the form of tofu, soy milk, miso, soy flour and so on is a major contributor to these remarkable health statistics.

What about soy gives Asian women this edge? The extraordinary compounds found in soy work as impressive antioxidants, inhibit the action of certain damaging compounds, help to normalize cell replication, keep hormones like estrogen from binding to breast tissue, lower cholesterol and have significant anti-tumor activity. Including soy in a diet that also emphasizes fresh fruits and vegetables, as well as whole grains, is vital to not only maintaining good health but also warding off a number of potentially fatal diseases as well.

Another reason why soy foods have received such intense interest is because they are considered the only nutritionally significant dietary source of compounds called isoflavones (in addition to being a source of high quality protein that is low in fat and high in omega-3 fatty acids). These properties are essential to soy's effectiveness. In fact, soy is the perfect example of Mother Nature's genius. Its wonderful array of phytonutrients work synergistically to protect the body from cancer and prompt overall health.

The Joy of Soy

The Chinese have known for centuries what we are just beginning to appreciate: the soybean (*ta-tou*), which means greater bean, was a food to be treated with respect. Considered sacred to Asian cultures, which have long recognized its therapeutic and life-sustaining properties, the soybean has been a staple of the Asian diet. Soy dates back prior to 2000 B.C., as recorded in Chinese literature, and found its way into Japan in the sixth century A.D. Europeans became acquainted with soy in the seventeenth century, and although Americans have known about soy for decades, it has only been in recent years that scientific data has surfaced to support its extraordinary nutritive value. Ironically, although the United States supplies one-third of the world's total soybean production, it pays the least attention to soy. According to the U.S. Department of Agriculture, soybean production in the United States totaled 2.38 billion bushels in 1996. Soybean production represented the third largest crop, behind corn and wheat in the United States. However, most of America's soybean crop is promptly exported to other countries. Of additional interest is the view of University of Illinois' researcher Michael Plewa, who believes that because we produce so much soy, we have the opportunity to discover new therapeutic compounds in soy leftovers, which are cast aside after soybean oil or soy meal is produced.

Soy comes in over 1,000 varieties and ranges in size from a small pea to as large as a grape. The soybean can be red, yellow, green, brown or black and has a rather bland taste. While technically a member of the legume family, the soybean differs from other beans in that it's low in carbohydrates and high in protein. Most of us have probably seen soy as tofu (soybean curd), soybean oil, soy flour, soy milk, soy sauce or miso. New soy foods are currently hitting the world market at a rapid rate, attesting to soy's impressive versatility.

Most Americans don't know that soy extracts are commonly used in margarines, salad oils, coffee creamers, meat substitutes, etc., for their texturing effects. Unfortunately, these soy sources fail to provide us with enough of soy's phytonutrients to really make a difference. Whole soy foods need to comprise a much greater percentage of our dietary intake, even though, to date, they have played a rather inconsequential role in our diets.

Super Protein Source

The soybean is considered a complete food because it contains protein, carbohydrates and fat, as well as an impressive array of minerals including calcium and iron. Soybeans have the distinction of being the only vegetable source of complete protein. Protein is essential for our bodies' various regenerative processes, and it helps to transport oxygen to our cells while fortifying our immune defenses. Eating an excess of animal protein, rather than vegetable protein, is one reason that many Americans suffer from cholesterol-related diseases and certain cancers.

A complete protein contains all eight essential amino acids, which cannot be produced by the body and must come from a dietary source. Meat and eggs contain complete proteins but can pose health risks if eaten in excess. Remarkably, soy contains this vital array of amino acids without any of the drawbacks of animal protein foods. In fact, soy has been designated as a protein alternative that is considered equal to meat. All of us, with the exception of infants, who need additional methionine, could exist on soy as our single source of protein if we had (or wanted) to.

The soybean supplies us with even more protein than an equivalent amount of cheese, milk, eggs or even fish but contains no cholesterol or saturated fat. In other words, the soybean is high quality vegetable protein—better for us than meat and much less expensive to produce ounce per ounce. Given the newly adopted guidelines for rating proteins, the FDA now gives soy the highest possible protein score.

Soy also contains calcium, phosphorus, iron, magnesium, thiamine, riboflavin and niacin. (With the exception of tempeh, however, it is not a good source of vitamin B12, which is one reason why vegetarians are often advised to use B12 supplementation.) Besides the many benefits soy offers to women, soy can also help reduce blood pressure, regulate blood sugar, promote better bowel function, lower cholesterol, strengthen bones, protect against various cancers, balance out hormones, boost immunity and protect cells as an antioxidant.

Soy Mania

As scientists become aware of the soy compounds that have the most profound protective properties, attention is directed toward how quickly these chemicals can be isolated, genetically engineered and marketed as both food supplements and medicines. Because soy has emerged from relative obscurity, separating soy fact from fiction is crucial in order to assess its true capabilities. Inevitably, more studies will continue to appear as researchers in Western medicine validate what Asian cultures have known for millennia. Soy's impact on breast cancer has to be one of its most dramatic properties. Soy compounds can actually manipulate estrogen in the female body, and estrogen plays a major role in the development of breast cancer.

Breast Cancer, Estrogen Levels and Soy

Remember that when a cell's delicate cycle malfunctions, the cell may become unable to turn off its reproductive mechanisms, resulting in the formation of a tumor. The question of why this occurs involves the possible influence of many factors. When it comes to breast cancer, however, the role of estrogen is prime. When estrogen hooks up with a receptor cite in breast tissue, it can stimulate cell division. In fact, some evidence suggests that estrogen actually accelerates the cell cycle, which can cause uncontrolled growth in breast, prostate and uterine tissue—the primary estrogen receptor sites. So why are American women so vulnerable to this estrogen effect, while their Japanese sisters seem protected?

Scientists believe that the phytoestrogen content of soy may explain why the incidence of breast cancer in Japanese and Chinese women is only one-fifth that of Western women. The average intake of soy protein in Southeast Asia ranges from ten to fifty grams per day, contrasted with one to three grams consumed in the United States. The effect that soy has on estrogen in the human body may be the single most important reason why Asian women are at such a lower risk for breast cancer.

Remember that the longer your breast tissue is exposed to circulating estrogen, the greater your risk of growing a malignant tumor. A report of three separate studies on test groups out of the University of Texas Medical Branch in Galveston showed that women who drank soy milk had lower levels of estrogen in their blood. This finding was reported to a meeting of the American Association for Cancer Research (AACR) as another indicator supporting the idea that soy affords Asian women breast cancer protection. The test groups of six to ten women each were given thirty-five ounces of soy milk, or approximately four large glasses, daily for between one and five months. The estrogen levels in some of the women who drank soy milk were reduced 30–40 percent, dramatically illustrating the impressive estrogen-blocking action of soy. But before you run out and buy soy milk, read on— not all soy milk is created equal. A later section will discuss how to pick out the best soy products.

Soy's Anticancer Biochemistry

Unquestionably, as we mentioned earlier, soy is packed with anticancer compounds, including protease inhibitors, phytates, phytosterols, saponins and other agents that may also be cancer-protective, such as lecithin, the omega-3 essential fatty acids and phenolic acids. Bowman-Birk Inhibitor (BBI), contained in soy, has proven its ability to prevent and inhibit the formation of cancerous cells, with no toxic effects, in vitro (test tube studies) and in animal models as well. Another point of interest is that a concentrated and more potent form of BBI, called BBIC, has been given a designation of Investigational New Drug Status (IND no. 34671) and has been used in human trials for cancer prevention. Our discussion, however, will focus on soy compounds called isoflavones, which have the distinct ability to mimic human estrogen. Of all of nature's phytoestrogens, they are perhaps the most impressive.

chapter 4

The Power of Soy Isoflavones

"Nature never breaks her own laws."
LEONARDO DA VINCI

OVER THE LAST decade in particular, soy isoflavones have been the subject of intense research. As data emerges, more reasons surface as to why women should be asking their doctors about using isoflavones. Isoflavones are phytoestrogens that exert weak estrogenic activity and have other beneficial actions in the human body. While phytoestrogens can be found in other plants, the soybean is the richest source. Soybean isoflavones are approximately 500 to 1,000 times weaker in their activity than that of estradiol (a human form of estrogen), yet their impact in the body can be significant.

Soy's two primary isoflavones are called genistein and daidzein and their respective glucosides, genistin and daidzin. Genistein is the predominant phytoestrogen found in the outer portion of soybeans, while daidzein is found in the germ of the bean. You may have already seen isoflavone supplements in your local health food store, and we will discuss their pros and cons in a later section of this book.

Soy foods typically contain more genistein than daidzein, although this ratio can change depending on the type of soy food analyzed. Over 1,000 clinical studies prove that genistein acts as a weak estrogen in the body. Both genistein and daidzein have the remarkable ability to attach to receptor sites in breast and other tissue that would normally bind with estrogens made by the female body.

Consequently, isoflavones provide significant protection to vulnerable tissue that may form estrogen-stimulated cancers. In other words, isoflavones trick the body into thinking that its own estrogen has already been there. In this way, they act as "anti-estrogens." They can, however, also act paradoxically by stimulating mild estrogenic activity, which is why they are so valuable for postmenopausal women.

How Isoflavones Possess Both Estrogenic and Antiestrogenic Properties

The notion that a chemical can act to mimic estrogen and suppress or enhance its effects is enormously intriguing. The term selective estrogen receptor modulators (SERM) has been used to describe such compounds, which have all the good and none of the bad attributes of estrogen. Like estrogen, these modulators support cardiovascular and bone health, but in estrogen-sensitive tissues like in the breast, they actually block the negative effects of circulating estrogen. As far as soy goes, it is now also thought that soy isoflavones not only mimic estrogen but may also stimulate the production of a compound called sex hormone binding globulin (SHBG), which makes estrogen less potent.

Dr. Kenneth Setchell of the Children's Hospital and Medical Center in Cincinnati, Ohio, a well-known soy expert, actually identified a phytoestrogen called "equol" in the urine of people who had consumed soy. He states, "These bioactive non-nutrients are strikingly similar in chemical structure to estradiol, the main female hormone. Indeed, one can superimpose almost exactly the structures of estradiol and isoflavones so they become indistinguishable, and therefore they fit beautifully into the pocket representing the binding domain of the estrogen receptor." Moreover, Dr. Setchell emphasizes that these isoflavones also possess many other important nonhormonal properties that have made them the subject of intense research.

Simply stated, isoflavones are nonsteroidal estrogens that are amazingly similar in their chemical structure to female estrogens but not identical. They can act as estrogens, which is what you want if you're menopausal, or they can antagonize estrogens, which works to decrease PMS and breast cancer risk. For example, if a woman has had a hysterectomy or has passed through menopause, she will produce very little estrogen. In this case, isoflavones can actually link up to open estrogen receptor sites on cells and produce a weak estrogen effect. On the other hand, for those women who suffer from an estrogen dominance, isoflavones compete with natural estrogen for receptor sites, thereby decreasing the estrogenic effect responsible for PMS and other related problems.

American Women and Isoflavones

Typically, an Asian woman receives thirty to eighty milligrams (two to three ounces) of soy isoflavones per day by eating tofu, miso, natto, tempeh, etc. By contrast, American women are lucky to get one or two milligrams of isoflavones daily, which they unknowingly consume as soy protein used in processed foods. Realistically, few American women eat the amounts of soy they should—a fact that reflects the tenacity of food biases we grew up with. Interestingly, Asian women who come to America and exchange their traditional eating habits for American ones also exchange their chances for developing breast cancer. In other words, when Asian women start eating like their American sisters, the protection they once enjoyed disappears—showing that the cancer risk is not completely genetic.

Asian-Americans and Breast Cancer

Unfortunately, American-born children of Asian immigrants have a 60 percent higher risk of developing breast cancer than do people born in Asia. Studies reveal shocking differences in cancer rates between Asians living in Asia and their relatives in America. One study, which looked at breast cancer among Chinese, Japanese and Filipino American women living in Los Angeles, San Francisco and Oahu, found that intake of tofu was more than twice as high among Asian-American women born in Asia as compared with those born in the United States. Among immigrants, intake of tofu decreased with years of residence in the United States. The study found that risk of breast cancer decreased when tofu consumption increased in both pre- and postmenopausal women. This study powerfully points out the importance of daily soy consumption for continuing protection. If you stop, your risk escalates.

The Overall Effects of Isoflavones

We've briefly talked about soy isoflavones and how they act as weak estrogens. Let's look at all the health-promoting properties of soy isoflavones that set them apart as one of nature's most remarkable phytonutrients. According to peer-reviewed scientific studies, soy can do the following:

• prevent cancer at multiple sites with cancer enzyme inhibitors
• act as estrogens and antiestrogens (to help with menopausal and PMS symptoms)
• prevent gallstones
• protect kidney functions

- stimulate bone formation (to help protect the bones from osteoporosis)
- lower cholesterol levels
- inhibit the oxidation of LDL cholesterol
- inhibit the development or progression of atherosclerosis
- act as powerful antioxidants
- enhance immune function

Genistein: Star Isoflavone

Soybeans are the single most significant dietary source of genistein—which is considered the most important soy isoflavone. Genistein was identified in 1966 but did not come to the forefront of scientific recognition until the 1970s. The more researchers learned about genistein, the more scientific buzz was generated.

At a recent international symposium on soy, genistein was the subject of various clinical studies. Herman Adlercreutz, M.D., Ph.D., of the Department of Clinical Chemistry at the University of Helsinki was in attendance and is considered one of the world's leading experts on genistein. One of the most exciting developments presented at the symposium was the work of a University of Alabama researcher who revealed the first in vivo (living subject) evidence that genistein retards cancer development.

His study exposed newborn female rats to a carcinogen that stimulates the growth of breast tumors. The rats were then either given an inactive compound or genistein. All of the rats receiving the inactive compound developed tumors. By contrast, only 60 percent of the rats receiving genistein developed cancer. This was the first study done in live animals showing that genistein can protect against chemically induced breast cancer. Scores of other in vitro (test tube) studies done since then have supported genistein's ability to inhibit tumor growth, as well.

How Genistein Helps Prevent Cancer

Genistein targets various stages of cancer development in a variety of ways. In other words, genistein can modify the way cells reproduce by targeting certain proteins. It can actually alter certain chemical pathways responsible for creating out-of-control cell growth, and it can also block the blood and nutrient supply needed by a tumor to keep growing. What is particularly impressive is that genistein can accomplish these effects through oral ingestion. Its actions are not destroyed by the digestive process. A paper presented at the National Pharmacy Week Celebration in 1997 reported that there are a number of ways that genistein functions to reduce the risk of cancer.

1. Genistein has only 1/1,000 the hormonal activity of estrogen, attaches to the breast cells' estrogen receptors, and by doing so keeps the more potent and potentially dangerous female hormone from attaching to estrogen receptors.

2. It is now known that genistein may decrease hypothalamic and pituitary gland activity which causes the ovaries to produce less estrogen. Tests have found that premenopausal women who ate an isoflavone-rich diet (45 milligrams/day for one month) increased the length of their cycles, which delayed menstruation. Remember that the longer a woman's cycle is, the fewer cycles she will have over a lifetime—this results in less exposure for estrogen-sensitive breast tissue.

3. Genistein causes mammary glands to become more mature and cells to become more diverse, thereby protecting tissue against the formation of tumors. For women who have never nursed, this is significant because their glands stay immature, and they are more vulnerable to tumor formation.

4. Genistein functions as a powerful antioxidant, which also contributes to its anticancer effects. It is capable of scavenging for oxygen-reactive free radicals that can initiate mutations in

breast and other tissue. Genistein may also increase the amount of superoxide dismutase (SOD), a powerful antioxidant that helps to stop the damage caused by superoxide radicals, produced in the body. Another fascinating discovery at the Mount Sinai School of Medicine in New York reported that genistein also seems to act as an SOD imitator. In addition, a study published in a 1997 issue of Free Radical Research describes genistein as the most powerful antioxidant isoflavone (followed by daidzein). Remember that antioxidant compounds are considered significant cancer-protective agents.

5. Genistein also inhibits two biochemicals, called tyrosine kinase and topoisomerase II, which play a very significant role in cell reproduction and have been linked to the formation of many cancers. Over and over, laboratory trials have consistently shown that genistein is capable of inhibiting the activity of tyrosine kinase. Some of the most powerful chemotherapy drugs we use today have been designed to do the same thing. In light of this data, genistein appears to act not only as a cancer-protector but may also be beneficial if you already have cancer.

6. Genistein contributes to programmed cell death, which works to regulate tumor cell growth. Imagine what would happen if cells reproduced themselves without the normal controls. Researchers now believe that genistein helps to stop tumor cell growth by stimulating this mechanism.

7. Genistein inhibits a process called angiogenesis, which is the generation of new capillaries to feed solid tumors, so that they become nutrient-starved and shrink. Tests reveal that genistein is the most potent of several plant compounds that prevent the growth of blood vessels in new tumors, which can stop tumor growth. Pharmaceutical companies are in the process of designing powerful drugs that can accomplish what Mother Nature has already given us. In fact, you may have already seen magazine advertisements touting new estrogenic drugs

that use soy isoflavones in their blend. Be aware that these are still forms of synthetic hormones.

8. Genistein helps to prevent multidrug resistance to anticancer drugs. This phenomenon leads to the failure of cancer chemotherapy due to decreased drug accumulation in resistant cells. Laboratory studies have shown that genistein is capable of reversing decreased drug accumulation. One study has found that genistein can decrease the resistance of leukemia cells to a number of anticancer drugs.

9. Genistein suppresses the production of harmful stress proteins. Scientists at the University of Southern California School of Medicine found that genistein helps to inhibit the action of proteins that help cancer cells to escape destruction by the immune system. Dr. Amy S. Lee, one of the authors of the study which was published in the *Journal of the National Cancer Institute,* believes that genistein is a potent inhibitor of cell proliferation that can suppress the growth of cancers in rats and human leukemia cells transplanted into mice.

10. One fascinating action of genistein is that it appears to transform some malignant cells into benign cells, which puts a halt to the cancer process on the cellular level. More studies are needed to explore this mechanism.

11. Genistein may stop the movement of cancer cells from one place to another. Researchers at Nebraska's Creighton University School of Medicine in Omaha conducted a study that found that soy could dramatically reduce the movement of cancer cells within the body from one site to another (metastasis). In this study, the spread of cancer cells and the number of developing tumors significantly decreased among 45 soy-fed mice.

(*Note:* In a study published in 1997, daidzein, another soy isoflavone, emerged as a significant immune enhancer that may reduce the risk of cancer, due to its ability to stimulate lymphocyte activity in a way that genistein alone could not. This suggests that the two compounds should be consumed together as nature intended for maximum effect.)

We can't think of a plant nutrient that has a more impressive list of cancer-preventing properties than genistein—which lends more validity to why all of us should be eating foods made from soybeans. Soy's effectiveness against breast cancer is one of its primary benefits; however, another use of isoflavones (like genistein) that is now in the spotlight and deserves discussion is its use in conjunction (or in place of) HRT for menopausal women. The subject of HRT is especially important when talking about breast cancer risks because of the recent debate over how the therapies are actually manipulating cancer risks in women, if at all. In the next chapter, we will discuss the benefits and drawbacks of HRT and soy for women going through the hormone changes associated with menopause and how these therapies may be used together.

chapter 5

Hormone Replacement Therapy vs. Soy

"I will follow that system of regimen which, according to my ability and judgement, I consider for the benefit of my patients, and abstain from whatever is deleterious."

FROM THE HIPPOCRATIC OATH

FOR WOMEN, DECIDING whether to take hormone replacement therapy (HRT)—formerly referred to as estrogen replacement therapy (ERT)—or not can be a very difficult decision. There is a compelling list of pros and cons, and to make matters worse, clinical studies often arrive at opposite conclusions, only adding to the confusion. Frequently, when making this decision, women rely on others' preferences and experience rather than facts because the "facts" are so contradictory. Research out of Harvard Medical School in Boston reveals that women who were already on HRT had decided to take the drugs primarily due to opinions expressed by their medical providers, the media and their friends. In fact, according to a report in the *British Journal of General Practice,* only 5 percent of women who were on HRT had requested it from their doctor.

A better way for women to make this very important decision is for them to consider their own preferences, needs and experience. Before deciding to use HRT, women should weigh all the pluses and minuses for their specific situation and then make an educated choice. Many women ask us if HRT is safe, but there is no definitive answer to that question yet. Some studies suggest that the dangers of HRT are minimal while others warn against its long-term use. Naturally, whenever a synthetic hormone is administered in drug form, there is a reasonable cause for concern. In this chapter, we will explore all the options available and examine why soy can play a very important role for women who have had hysterectomies or are postmenopausal, whether they choose to use HRT or not.

The Risks of Estrogen Depletion

When a patient asks us what will happen if she does not use any kind of hormone therapy after menopause, we advise her that some form of estrogen replacement (natural or artificial) is usually warranted since estrogen depletion can contribute to brittle bones, heart disease and even some types of premature senility. Replenishing the female body with safe forms of estrogen after menopause seems like a good idea—whether or not HRT falls into the safe category is still the subject of intense debate. We have to admit, however, that the notion of taking hormones indefinitely after menopause seems completely unnatural.

If nature meant for women's bodies to make estrogens and progesterones until they die, why does menopause even exist? Also, not all women may need estrogen replacement after menopause. Our primary concern, then, is the rampant dispersal of synthetic hormones to women—even women who have a low risk for osteoporosis and heart disease. Each woman has her own set of needs based on her inherited risks and hormone levels, and by passing out one solution and saying it works for every woman, medical professionals are not only being too simplistic in their solution but also reckless. The hormone solution a woman chooses should be as individual as the woman. That is the beauty and great advantage that natural phytoestrogens offer—they are a no-risk way to tackle the dilemma of women's varying hormonal needs.

A Crash Course in Synthetic Hormonal Drugs

Conventional hormonal replacement therapy has various names, depending on the hormones it uses. ERT refers to drug therapies that consist of estrogen only. Progestin/estrogen replacement therapy (PERT) refers to drugs which use both estrogen and progesterone. Other ERT drugs, such as Raloxifene, have recently been approved for use and claim to have lower potential risk factors. Despite claims, however, that these drugs are safe, they have since been linked to an increased risk for ovarian cancer.

Another drug recently investigated for its bone-protecting ability in postmenopausal women is Alendronate (or Fosamax). It was found to prevent bone loss in women under the age of 60 almost to the same extent as estrogen/progestin. However, it also has produced side effects, such as severe esophageal inflammation, in some women.

The most common form of estrogen prescribed in this country is conjugated estrogen, which is sold under the brand name of Premarin. Estrace is also used and is actually made from yam extracts, which are natural phytoestrogens, but it is still artificially synthesized in the laboratory. Premarin is produced from pregnant mares' urine and is called conjugated equine estrogen, which is a mixture of various estrogenic compounds. This form of hormone replacement therapy has been the source of much scientific debate.

HRT Delivery Systems: Pros and Cons

Approximately 15–20 percent of all postmenopausal women currently use some form of ERT. Although all forms of HRT have received mixed reviews, most physicians will agree that conjugated estrogen can significantly reduce heart disease and osteoporosis in postmenopausal women. The key to minimizing the possible side effects of HRT seems to lie in its dosage—the least possible therapeutic dose is the most desirable.

Long ago, estrogen prescriptions were routinely given at 1.25 milligrams to 2.5 milligrams per day. Today, doctors prescribe a daily dose of 0.625 milligrams. Also, if you choose to use HRT, your doctor will discuss oral preparations versus patches placed directly on the skin. Some of these drugs are taken daily while others are taken only on specific days of the month. Patches, however, have been associated with fewer side effects since they enter the bloodstream rather than taking the digestive route.

The Potential Risks of HRT: What to Believe

There are scores of studies on various aspects of HRT. Some studies have concluded that its use may increase the life expectancy of women, while others report that it reduces the risk of postmenopausal heart disease and osteoporosis. And still other studies show that it helps to prevent excessive wrinkling and keeps aging skin more supple. On the other hand, HRT has been linked to an increased risk for breast cancer as well as blood clots.

The truth is, no study is flawless, and no set of conclusions is without flaw. Some studies may be too observational; others may be too short-term or biased. Still others may not have a large enough or diverse enough sample. Because of these variables, contradictory data abounds. For example, one study will tell you that HRT reduces the risk for postmenopausal heart attack, while another says just the opposite.

Researchers from eighteen medical centers in the United States studied 2,763 postmenopausal women with known heart disease who were followed for an average of four years. The study was recently published in the *Journal of the American Medical Association (JAMA)*. The authors concluded that women taking active hormones actually had a 50 percent increase in their risk for a heart attack during the first year of treatment. What does this suggest? Obviously if there are cardiovascular benefits to HRT, these scientists believe they don't occur during the initial phase of therapy. HRT's benefits are balanced with its flaws.

Breast Cancer Risks and HRT

The breast cancer connection to HRT is just as confusing and inconclusive. More than thirty observational studies on breast cancer and HRT have yielded inconsistent results—cumulatively, these studies show a reduced risk, no risk or increased risk of breast cancer with synthetic hormone therapy.

One study conducted in Sweden claimed that women taking estrogen therapy may quadruple their risk of developing breast cancer. Women in the study who took a combination of estrogen and synthetic progestin for more than six years were 4.4 times more likely to develop breast cancer. Ironically, the progestin is added to estrogen therapy to help decrease the risk of developing uterine cancer, and in this study, it was the combination of estrogen and progestin that showed the highest risk of breast cancer. In fact, one study published in a 1994 issue of *Molecular and Cellular Endocrinology* reported that synthetic progestins induce the proliferation of breast tumor cells. It is important to consider various factors in these studies, including how the hormone therapy was administered, the route of administration, possible side effects, as well as how long it went on, before being able to adequately understand the full picture.

New Dangers of Progestins in HRT

The North American Menopause Society surveys show that about a third of American women ages forty-five to sixty-five—

some sixteen million women—use hormone supplements, either estrogen alone or a combination drug containing progestin. A study from the National Institutes of Health published in a year 2000 edition of *JAMA* reported that menopausal women using commonly prescribed hormone supplements that include a mix of estrogen and progestin run a 20 percent higher risk of breast cancer than those who take estrogen alone. To make matters more confusing, previous studies have linked some HRT drugs that include estrogen alone with higher rates of breast cancer. Adding to these are the studies concluding that neither progestin nor estrogen are associated with an increased risk of breast cancer. These conflicting results have prompted physicians to recommend that women proceed with caution when deciding whether to take HRT or not. In other words, ask questions before you fill that prescription.

The *JAMA* study collected data on hormone use from questionnaires given to 46,355 women who participated in a nationwide breast cancer screening project from 1980 through 1995. During this time, the survey cited 2,082 cases of breast cancer. Interestingly, compared with women who had never used synthetic hormones, women who had taken estrogen supplements within the previous four years had a 20 percent higher risk of developing breast cancer. For those women who were currently taking or had taken estrogen/progestin supplements, the risk was 40 percent higher than for nonusers. Moreover, the study found that for each year of use, the risk of developing breast cancer increased 1 percent for estrogen-only users and 8 percent for estrogen-progestin users. Women who had stopped taking either type of HRT for more than four years faced no increased risk, regardless of how long they had taken synthetic hormones. The study suggested that the body mass index of a woman must also be considered a factor in assessing risk as well as the type of HRT supplement.

This study motivated three Harvard University doctors, Walter Willett, Graham Colditz and Meir Stampfer, to publically call for further study on the long-term use of both hormones. These doctors have said that new questions on the safety of both synthetic

HOW TO MAKE AN INFORMED DECISION

Considering all the potential risks and benefits of estrogen replacement, we suggest that doctors and health professionals tell their patients that every woman must come to her own decision based on what is right for her alone. Each woman needs to consider her individual risk for osteoporosis, heart disease and breast cancer in order to make an appropriate choice. A woman will also need to consider the drawbacks associated with different therapies. For instance, synthetic estrogen used alone has been associated with fluid retention, increased fat storage, depression, headaches, impaired blood sugar control, gallbladder problems, decreased sex drive and ironically, possible fibroids and bone loss.

The attempt to offset the negative effects of estrogen replacement with synthetic progestins comes with additional hazards. Synthetic progestins have been linked with an increased risk of birth defects, liver dysfunction, breast tenderness, acne, insomnia, swelling and weight changes.

In truth, it makes sense to stay as close to nature as possible, even if using a synthetic preparation. In other words, if you choose to use HRT after a hysterectomy or menopause, select a drug formula that mimics what your body would produce, and use it in the lowest possible therapeutic dosage, which renders you protective benefits. If you are on HRT, you may want to gradually decrease your dosage until you are off of synthetic hormones, and then use plant estrogens like soy as a replacement for your previous therapy. Always talk to your doctor or health care provider before making any big changes.

estrogen and estrogen/progestin therapy warrant the use of other treatments. In a January 25, 2000 issue of *USA Today*, they stated, "The commonly held belief that aging routinely requires pharmacological management has unfortunately led to neglect of diet and lifestyle as the primary means to achieve healthy aging." We could not agree more and have cited soy isoflavones as a possible alternative to synthetic hormone replacement therapy.

Using Dietary Soy Instead of HRT

Surprisingly, it is estimated that over 80 percent of all post-menopausal women do not use any type of HRT. In light of this statistic, Gregory L. Burke, a medical doctor at the Bowman Gray School of Medicine at Wake Forest University, has studied the possibility of using dietary soy as a natural form of post-menopausal HRT. Keep in mind that we have already established the fact that replenishing estrogen after menopause is a good idea. According to Dr. Burke, the potential for dietary soy supplementation to serve as an alternative to HRT has been documented in both animal studies and even in some human clinical trials.

He cited a double-blind clinical trial of fifty-one women who were given soy protein isolate for a six-week period. Improvements in menopausal symptoms, as well as blood pressure and cholesterol profiles, were noted. Moreover, none of the negative side effects associated with synthetic HRT occurred. Dr. Burke stated, "If our studies turn out to be very positive in prevention of chronic disease and prevention of menopausal symptoms, we think [soy] is a wonderful alternative for many women."

Christine Conrad, co-author of *Natural Woman Natural Menopause*, which was published in 1997, states that soy isoflavones and other plant estrogens can be effective hormone replacement agents for women who have had hysterectomies. Dr. J. Koudy Williams, D.V.M. at the Bowman Gray School of Medicine said in light of his findings on the heart-protective properties of soy, "A dietary supplement [of soy] potentially may provide a viable alternative to traditional [estrogen] hormone replacement therapy."

It only stands to reason that if our goal is to re-create estrogenic effects in the female body after they have ceased, it is more effective to do it in a way that the body recognizes as user-friendly rather than adversarial. Soy isoflavones may offer women just such an option. And in fact, a recent study by Dr. T. Clarkson at Wake Forest University on using soy phytoestrogens instead of

HRT concluded that because current forms of HRT have a low acceptance rate among postmenopausal women, soy phytoestrogens may be the alternative natural option they have been looking for.

How Powerful Is the Estrogenic Effect of Soy Isoflavones?

If you are worried that soy isoflavones may not be strong enough to give you the same benefit as HRT, consider this: Dr. Kenneth D. Setchell, an expert on soy isoflavones, has found that after we eat soy isoflavones, they are metabolized by intestinal bacteria, absorbed from the intestinal tract and then transported to the liver. Remember that isoflavones are eliminated in the urine through the kidneys. He believes that even consuming modest amounts of soy protein results in relatively high circulating concentrations of phytoestrogens.

What his study suggests is that a consistent consumption of dietary soy will eventually cause a steady state of phytoestrogen levels in the blood. His research found that consuming quantities of soy-foods containing in the region of 50 milligrams per day of total isoflavones (close to what the Japanese traditionally consume) maintained these significant levels of phytoestrogens. This study suggests that soy consumption could very easily exert a significant hormonal effect in the female body. Dr. Setchell points out that what is considered an optimal dose of isoflavones remains to be established. He suggests that premenopausal women use amounts of soy consistent with that of people in countries where soy is consumed as a staple to obtain the same endocrine effects.

Using Soy with HRT: Reducing Health Risks

We believe it only makes sense that a diet which contains soy may be of benefit to anyone on traditional HRT. Naturally, moderation is the key, but there is a great deal of scientific support behind the notion of increasing your intake of phytoestrogenic foods in your menopausal years. Plus, soy not only contains phytoestrogens but also provides us with an impressive array of other marvelous phytonutrients. These marvelous compounds have proven their ability to protect the human body from a number of diseases, including cancer.

Although there is still much to learn about soy's potential to work as a safe HRT, soy's phytoestrogenic activity is very real. In addition, if taken in whole food form, dietary soy is infinitely safer than synthetic drug preparations. The key is learning to use soy consistently and listening to the needs of your own body. Moreover, if you decide that conventional HRT is best for you, follow the hormonal health guidelines listed in a later chapter to help mitigate the adverse effects of synthetic drugs. Of course, always check with your doctor before making any changes.

HRT: The Bottom Line

We believe that the message to postmenopausal women is clear. Women should not be ostracized if they choose to forgo traditional HRT. All the available data strongly suggests that using soy foods is a safer and less expensive way to stimulate estrogenic effects. Granted, it may not be as strong or pronounced in its influence, but this is actually one of its advantages as well. At the very least, women should be made aware that phytoestrogens like soy offer them a previously unknown option—an alternative to prescription hormones. Data suggests that the health risks of using conjugated estrogens and progestins, coupled with their high cost, should compel every woman to evaluate the possibility of using soy isoflavones as a potential alternative to pharmaceutical solutions.

The fact that soy isoflavones not only help to control undesirable hormonally-related symptoms but also simultaneously reduce the risk of the very cancers that are killing thousands of women makes soy a premium source of nutrition for all women. Something as simple as consuming forty to fifty milligrams of isoflavones daily may be enough to obtain the kind of results you need—and it isn't as hard as you may think.

Scientists at the National Institute of Environmental Health Sciences conducted a study with postmenopausal women who were given a variety of soy-based foods for sixty days. Soy nuts, soy spreads, soy milk, tofu and related items were used, and the number of isoflavones consumed by each woman was estimated to be over two hundred milligrams. What this study suggests is that it may be easier to consume desired levels of isoflavones, by using a variety of soy foods, than most of us thought (refer to the recipe chapter).

If you have had your ovaries removed and are experiencing premature menopause, you may need to use a combination of estrogen replacement and dietary soy supplementation. If you feel that you need a prescription form of HRT, look for new varieties that are using soy and yam compounds to synthesize the original synthetic drug compounds.

It is also important to remember that soy supplementation is not just for those looking to go off of HRT; it can also be helpful for pre- and perimenopausal women and can help with such issues as PMS, irregular periods, cramping, fatigue, infertility, hormonally triggered depression, weight gain and acne, as well as hot flashes and other menopausal symptoms. In addition, balancing hormone levels well before menopause may be a factor in preventing bone and heart problems and cancer risks by reducing excess amounts of circulating estrogen before they cause a problem. In the next chapter, we will discuss exactly how soy can be used to remedy the complications of PMS and menopause.

chapter 6

Menopause and PMS

*"It is not good to know more unless we do
more with what we already know."*

R.K. BERGETHON

DECADES AGO, PMS used to be called "premenstrual tension" and was considered a rather dubious disorder by most medical doctors. Today we know that PMS is a real problem for thousands of women and that it is caused by hormonal fluctuations. It certainly qualifies as the most common endocrine disorder seen in the industrialized world. While the onset of a menstrual period usually brings relief, many woman have noticed that they seem to have more bad days during their monthly cycle than good ones. Obviously, PMS is a multifaceted syndrome that is controlled by progesterone/estrogen relationships.

Premenstrual syndrome refers to a variety of symptoms initiated by hormonal factors that occur two to fourteen days before the onset of a period. Symptoms usually start around mid-cycle and reach their peak during the last seven days before menstruation. Once a period has begun, symptoms usually subside. The symptoms of PMS vary with each individual and typically get worse with age, due to declining progesterone levels. It has always been our view that PMS is directly linked with unopposed estrogen or an estrogen overload. Our experience is that most women report more than one of the following symptoms:

- acne
- bloating
- headache
- changes in sexual desire
- difficulty concentrating
- irritability

- backache
- fatigue
- sore or enlarged breasts
- depression
- difficulty coping with life
- tearfulness

Physicians Frequently Fail to Successfully Treat PMS

We know firsthand that PMS greatly compromises the quality of life for thousands of women who struggle to cope with this recurring and often worsening syndrome. Recent statistics report that at least 40 percent of all women between the ages of fourteen and fifty experience PMS. The emotional impact of this disorder is perhaps the most troubling and can cause heightened tension bad enough to jeopardize even the best of relationships. PMS is commonly misdiagnosed, and even when it's recognized, it is often poorly treated.

A recent survey published in the September 1998 issue of the *Journal of Women's Health* involving 220 women between the ages of twenty-six and fifty-six tells us that 64 percent of the women expressed dissatisfaction with their current therapies for PMS. The study concluded that "physicians from whom most of the women sought care between 1974 and 1994 failed to recognize, diagnose or treat their PMS using the standards and protocols published in the medical literature." Only a minority of physicians used a symptom chart to assess their patients' conditions, and only approximately one in four (26 percent) of physicians provided a helpful treatment. Seventy-six percent of subjects reported that their PMS diagnosis came initially from them, with a later agreement by the physician. Eighty-one percent reported that the initial suggestion that they may be PMS sufferers came from a nonmedical source—these are not flattering statistics for the medical profession.

PMS: An Estrogen Escapade Gone Bad

Because PMS is usually at its worst one week prior to the onset of the period when progesterone levels drop, the notorious estrogen factor again emerges. It's no coincidence that the word estrogen is derived from the Greek *oistros*, meaning "mad desire." Few women realize that they have estrogen receptors in the brain. The connection of the brain with estrogen explains the powerful emotional impact estrogen can have. Many women find that PMS worsens as they get older, suggesting that estrogen levels have become and remain imbalanced. Remember that hormone imbalances are more likely the closer a woman gets to menopause. How severe PMS is may also depend on genetics, diet, stress and whether or not a woman takes synthetic hormones.

The impact of hormonally fattened beef and dairy products is thought to play a role. Cows bred for milk production are routinely given hormones to increase their output, and animals bred for meat consumption often receive hormone injections to boost their market weight. In addition, a diet high in sugar, caffeine and hydrogenated fats is also thought to aggravate the problem. We now know that estrogen, serotonin (a brain chemical), appetite and depression are intrinsically linked, which sheds new light on the mechanics of PMS. We also know that even if your estrogen levels are declining as you age, so is your progesterone output, putting you at greater risk for an estrogen dominance and all the miserable symptoms we talked about in chapter one.

Soy and PMS Relief

So how does a woman tackle PMS? Eating soy foods on a regular basis may help to alleviate many PMS symptoms. Dr. Kenneth Setchell conducted a study in which a group of young women were given sixty grams of textured soy protein daily. After four weeks, their monthly cycles were lengthened by two to five days. Remember that the longer your cycle is, the less estrogen exposure you will experience over the course of your cycling lifetime. Lower circulating levels of estrogen mean less PMS—it's that simple. This same study also assessed the effect of taking sixty grams of miso daily, which lengthened the cycle one additional day. Of equal interest is that this effect lasted for two to three more cycles in some of the women, even after they had discontinued the soy food supplementation.

When phytoestrogens from soy take the place of estrogen on receptor sites in the breast, ovaries and uterus, the result is a longer interval between menstrual periods. In Japan, the average menstrual cycle is thirty-two days; in the United States, it's twenty-six to twenty-nine days. Researchers in England have looked into this difference with a study that included adding sixty grams of soy protein to the diet of female test subjects and then removing the soy while monitoring their cycles. (Sixty grams of soy protein is equivalent to the amount in three quarters of a cup of soybeans.) As long as the soy was consumed, the cycles in these women averaged two and one half days longer than before, and when the soy stopped, their cycles returned to their pre-soy length.

Of equal interest is that this study discovered that it was the early pre-ovulatory phase of the cycle that was lengthened, which is when the body is exposed to less estrogen. This is important because it's during the post-ovulatory phase of the cycle when levels of estrogen and progesterone increase and breast cells are stimulated to grow and can mutate into cancerous cells. Simply stated, if you reduce the number of menstrual periods you have over the course of a lifetime, your risk of developing breast cancer is also less—couple that with the ability of soy to bump estrogen off breast receptor sites, and you have a powerful preventative effect.

Soy is also rich in magnesium, which has a positive effect on PMS. One study in particular found that a test group of women had lower than normal levels of red blood cell magnesium—which has also been linked to diseases like chronic fatigue and fibromyalgia that target women. (If you suffer from PMS, you may also be at a higher risk for osteoporosis.)

Other Tips for Easing PMS Symptoms

• Exercise on a regular basis. Exercise has numerous benefits for PMS sufferers. Exercise releases tension and raises endorphin levels, which help us to manage pain and feel better about life. Exercise is also an invaluable stress-reliever that can play a major role in easing PMS irritability and related symptoms.

• Eat nutritiously. A diet that is low in refined sugars and flours and high in fresh raw vegetables and fruits, whole grains, high quality protein and good fats (omega-3 and omega-9) can go a long way in treating PMS. In addition, add soy-protein to your diet, and get away from caffeinated drinks and sugared soda. We believe that PMS is one of many disorders spawned, at least in part, by poor eating habits, and we can experience at least some relief by making the proper dietary changes.

• Take supplemental vitamin B6. Some women report that 200 to 300 milligrams of vitamin B6 taken two weeks before their periods helps to alleviate some PMS symptoms.

• Extra calcium and magnesium can ease PMS symptoms. Taking supplemental calcium resulted in a 50 percent reduction of PMS symptoms in one clinical study of 400 women. Dr. Susan Thys-Jacobs of St. Lukes-Roosevelt Hospital reported that mood swings, tension, headaches and cramping were all alleviated with calcium supplementation. Food cravings also dropped by half, and water retention decreased by more than one-third.

Recommended dosages are to take at least 1,000 milligrams of calcium a day. Chewable tablets are also suggested.

• Use natural progesterone creams. These creams have natural compounds that are close in their chemical structure to progesterone and are absorbed through the skin. They can help to balance estrogen, thereby easing PMS. Recommended dosage is one half teaspoon of the cream applied twice daily for the last two weeks of your cycle on vascular areas where veins are visible. Many women have also told us that rubbing the cream between their thighs at bedtime was helpful; however, try varying the place of application often to keep skin sensitive to the hormone. Places of application include inner arm and behind the knees, among others. If you want more information on natural progesterone creams, refer to books by Dr. John R. Lee, who is considered one of the foremost experts on using these creams for women's disorders.

Menopause: How to Avoid the Pitfalls

Going through the "big change" has traditionally been regarded as an event to be dreaded by both women and their male companions. Most of us have heard horror stories about the impending and frightening transformations associated with the advent of menopause. Archaic attitudes toward the perils of menopause have done little to educate women (and men) accurately about this natural transition. Getting the right information is the best way to successfully deal with menopause in our youth-worshiping society.

Today, as the baby boomers head into their middle years, record numbers of women are facing menopause. The next two decades will see over forty million American women entering their forties and early fifties. There are now over seventeen million women over the age of fifty in the United States. As the year

2020 approaches, sixty million women will be experiencing or will have passed through menopause. Most of those women will live out at least twenty-five post-menopausal years. The secrets to managing menopause are rooted in prescriptions for good health, of which soy can play a major role. Ultimately, it is most important that menopause not be viewed as a disorder but as a perfectly natural event that women should not have to suffer through.

A Working Definition of Menopause

Technically speaking, menopause refers to the permanent cessation of menstruation. It is a Greek term that combines the words monthly and cease. It's important to remember, however, that menopausal symptoms can occur for several years before and after a woman's final period. Menopause is actually a three-part process that cumulatively ends the reproductive life of the human female.

The first phase of menopause is sometimes called perimenopause and can start as early as age thirty-five as estrogen levels begin to decline. Erratic changes in the length of the menstrual cycle and the amount of flow are common during these years, along with symptoms typical of PMS (breast tenderness, irritability, forgetfulness, mood swings etc.). In fact, some people have referred to menopause as nothing more than a bad case of PMS. For many women, this time interval can be the worst phase of the whole process. Frequently, women neglect to link their newfound symptoms to perimenopause, causing them to feel out of control and confused. For this very reason, properly anticipating menopause with good diet, nutritional supplements and exercise is critical. Women need to know what is happening to their bodies and recognize that their symptoms can be addressed. They need not suffer in silence.

In addition, while most of us understand that estrogen levels drop as we age, the role of progesterone has been significantly

WHEN DOES MENOPAUSE BEGIN?

Menopause can occur anytime between the ages of thirty-five and fifty-five, although fifty-two commonly signals the end of menstruation. Each woman who lives beyond the age of fifty-five will inevitably experience menopause, although various factors can determine its onset. Variables that can affect the advent of menopause include:

- Nutritional state. Menopause can begin much earlier in women who suffer from malnutrition.

- Smoking. It can initiate earlier menopause by one to two years.

- Early onset of periods. The earlier menstruation began, the more likely that menopause will begin later.

- Using birth control pills. Some evidence suggests that using birth control pills may delay the onset of menopause.

- Heredity. Women tend to inherit the menstrual patterns of their mothers and grandmothers.

neglected. Hormonal chain reactions triggered by menopause may also result in less progesterone which, in and of itself, can cause menstrual-cycle changes (increased PMS, moodiness, etc). Remember that hormone levels can wildly fluctuate during perimenopause, causing everything from migraine headaches to intense food cravings and early hot flashes.

When the ovaries fail to produce enough estrogen to trigger menstruation, menopause has technically begun and usually lasts for one year following the last period. After a year has passed with no menstruation, the final stage of menopause called postmenopause ensues. This particular phase continues until the end of life, which points out the fact that many women will belong to the postmenopausal category for at least one third of their lives.

Symptoms That Give Menopause Its Bad Name

Various symptoms are associated with the hormonal changes that accompany menopause. Many women, however, only experience mild discomfort. On the other hand, a significant number of women suffer symptoms severe enough to require medical attention. In this country, a majority of women only have hot flashes, while approximately 25 percent feel unusually fatigued or depressed. Regardless of the number or severity of the symptoms, they stem from the same source.

Reduced estrogen and progesterone levels and imbalances cause most menopausal symptoms. Because ovulation is altered as a woman ages, progesterone levels decline prior to menopause and therefore also before an estrogen decline. Progesterone production almost ceases to exist at all at this time, while estrogen production declines to around 50 percent. This fact only compounds the problem of an estrogen/progesterone imbalance and explains why women in perimenopause can still suffer from an estrogen dominance even when their estrogen levels are in decline.

The symptoms that most women typically complain of include:

- anxiety
- forgetfulness
- heart palpitations
- inability to concentrate
- joint pain
- moodiness
- skin dryness
- vaginal dryness
- fatigue
- headaches
- hot flashes
- insomnia
- loss of sexual desire
- night sweating
- urinary tract disorders
- weight gain

Hormonal fluctuations may throw off the body's thermostat, resulting in hot flashes or night sweats. Low estrogen levels can also produce less vaginal secretion, resulting in dry tissue—a condition that can be alleviated by using vaginal lubricants.

Estrogen, Food and Mood

The mental and emotional changes associated with menopause, however, are often the hardest to deal with. These changes occur because hormonal levels affect estrogen receptors in the brain. Studies conducted at the Laboratory of Neuroendocrinology at Rockefeller University in New York suggest that dropping estrogen levels may reduce the number of neuron connections in the brain, causing forgetfulness or mental fuzziness.

Hormonal fluctuations also impact serotonin, a brain chemical that powerfully influences mood. Pre- and postmenopausal women may suffer from low serotonin levels which explains, at least in part, their struggle with depression. If this is the case, these women may be chronic carbohydrate cravers as well. Eating carbohydrate foods helps to raise serotonin levels and explains why some women prone to depression can't seem to get enough carbohydrates.

The Wurtman study revealed that people who crave carbohydrates show a high susceptibility to clinical depression. In other words, if you have a tendency to binge on carbohydrate snacks, you may not be eating to satisfy true hunger. If you find yourself eating cookie after cookie or consuming half a bag of chips at one sitting, you may be a victim of a carbohydrate-related mood disorder, which can reflect a hormonal imbalance. When people who typically snacked this way were asked why they constantly ate foods they knew would create weight problems, they responded that they ate to combat tension, feelings of anxiety or mental fatigue. The result of eating several cookies or potato chips was the creation of a feeling of calmness and well being.

Further research at MIT has shown that some obese people use sugar or carbohydrates as a type of sedative to maintain this sense of well being. When their sugar levels drop, their feelings of anxiety return. Because estrogen surges profoundly impact not only our brain chemistry but blood sugar as well, you can see why some menopausal women gain weight so readily. Many women

MENOPAUSAL MYTHS

Despite the fact that good nutrition and exercise can enable a woman to remain active, attractive and healthy during her postmenopausal years, "the change" is still linked to all kinds of myths. Most women are aware of these menopausal tales of horror and tend to brace themselves for the event, anticipating the worse. Fortunately, any truth behind the archaic attitudes about menopause has all but vanished. The good news is that for many women, menopause can signal the beginning of a new and exciting phase of life, thanks to health advances and the accessibility of health and nutritional information. Here are some of the more common misconceptions associated with menopause:

• Menopause signals the end of sexuality.

• The hormonal chaos of menopause makes most women crazy.

• Weight gain is an inevitable consequence of menopause.

• Once menopause occurs, signs of aging (wrinkling, osteoporosis) always accelerate.

• Menopause signals the end of physical activity and fitness.

• Menopause is a marker of overall physical and mental decline.

are continually snacking in an attempt to elevate certain neurotransmitters in the brain that create sensations of security and contentment. What is important to realize is that studies like this indicate that when brain levels of serotonin increase, carbohydrate cravings decrease. Moreover, the Wurtman study also points out that in some people who have trouble with mood swings or PMS, the brain fails to respond as it should when starchy snacks are eaten; therefore, the craving persists and overeating occurs. Simply stated, when you normalize estrogen and progesterone ratios, you also help to stabilize brain chemistry and insulin levels. The result is better mood and more control over weight.

Japanese Women and Menopause

One very striking fact about Japanese women is that they seem to sail through menopause. Hot flashes and night sweats are virtually unheard of in Asian cultures. In fact, there is no Japanese word to describe a "hot flash." Again, the consumption of soy foods rich in phytoestrogens is thought to be directly linked with this phenomenon. Japanese women eat from 2.5 to 3.5 ounces of tofu per day, or thirty to fifty grams of soy protein, as opposed to the one to three grams consumed by women in the Unite States. One clinical study found that urinary excretion of isoflavonoids in Japanese women was 100–1,000 times higher than in American women, illustrating again why Japanese women report so few menopausal symptoms. The fact that hot flashes are uncommon in women from countries where the consumption of soy products is high cannot be dismissed as inconsequential.

Soy: Cure for Menopause?

At the Second International Symposium on the Role of Soy in Preventing and Treating Chronic Disease, which was held in Brussels, Belgium in September 1996, researchers reported the results of six human studies that looked at the benefits of soy for menopausal symptoms. Three of these studies found that a significant decrease in the incidence of hot flashes occurred with soy supplementation. The other studies also reported a slight improvement in menopausal symptoms and improvements in cholesterol, blood pressure and vaginal tissue. The forms of soy used in the studies included a soy protein isolate supplement, soy bars with forty milligrams of phytoestrogen and soy grits. In the three studies that reported significant improvements, including one conducted in Australia with fifty-eight postmenopausal women who reported a 40 percent reduction in hot flashes, female participants were consuming forty-five grams of soy flour per day over a twelve week period. Another trial conducted at the Royal Hospital for Women in Australia consisted of nine women who consumed 160 milligrams of isoflavones for twelve weeks and experienced a significant decrease in the number of hot flashes, from an average of 6.7 to 3.4 per day. Still another British study found that giving eighty milligrams of isoflavones to a group of women for two months resulted in a significant decrease in the number of hot flashes.

John Eden and an Australian team of researchers concluded that soy isoflavones are likely to be therapeutically beneficial for women with mild to moderate menopausal symptoms. And a more recent study conducted in Italy using 104 postmenopausal women reported a significant reduction in their number of hot flashes (45 percent versus 30 percent for the placebo substance) after twelve weeks. The group consumed sixty grams daily of soy protein isolate containing seventy-six milligrams of isoflavones.

Researchers at the Bowman Gray School of Medicine and Tufts University conducted an eighteen week study that looked at the effects of soy on forty-three women ages 45–55. For six weeks, the women added twenty grams (under one ounce, approximately two teaspoons) of powdered soy protein to their daily breakfast. For another six weeks, they added the same amount of soy protein to their diets but split the amount into two 10-gram doses. For a third six-week period, they added a look-alike powdered carbohydrate placebo to their diet. Significantly less severe hot flashes and night sweats were reported by those taking the soy. In addition, total cholesterol levels dropped an average of 10 percent without any of the side effects seen with conventional hormonal therapy.

How Much Soy Is Necessary to Prevent Hot Flashes?

It's easy to get confused when trying to decipher test results to come up with the ideal soy food for menopause and how much of it to eat. One to three servings of a recommended soy food (consult tables in a later section) should provide the right amount of isoflavones necessary to achieve positive results. Research still needs to be done to determine the optimal amount. Again, looking at what Asian women typically consume should be our guideline. The average Japanese woman eats three to four ounces of soy foods a day. That translates to a daily serving or two of tofu, tempeh or soy milk. Remember that it is the soy protein that contains the phytoestrogenic isoflavones. New evidence tells us that fifteen ounces of soy milk (about two cups) or two ounces of tofu daily might be all that a woman requires to control hot flashes and to help stabilize estrogen levels during menopause.

Guidelines for Relieving the Effects of Menopause

The following suggestions may help any premenopausal patient minimize menopausal symptoms:

- Do not smoke.
- Reduce caffeine intake. (Excess caffeine can leach calcium from the bones and cause breast fibroids.)
- Avoid alcohol and soft drinks.
- Eat plenty of fresh fruits and vegetables (at least five servings daily), and use high quality protein sources like soy foods and whole grains, emphasizing beans, legumes, raw nuts and seeds. Avoid sugary, fatty foods and meats, and remember that nutritional demands rise after menopause.
- Supplement the diet with appropriate nutrients (e.g., calcium and magnesium).
- Get regular aerobic and weight bearing exercise to prevent weight gain, osteoporosis and moodiness.
- Control blood sugar disorders to avoid the risk of heart disease.
- Wear light cotton, breathable fabrics, particularly at night if hot flashes are a problem.

- Consider using natural progesterone cream and phytoestrogenic herbs (discussed in a later chapter).
- Use a vaginal lubricant (Lubifax, K-Y) for vaginal dryness and itching. Other preparations that might be helpful are unscented creams.
- Drink plenty of water (at least four eight-ounce glasses daily) to help with hot flashes.
- Carry a packet of pre-moistened towelettes with you to cool off your face. Small battery operated fans are also helpful.
- Use relaxation techniques such as yoga or breathing exercises to combat anxiety and/or nervousness.

chapter 7

Isoflavones and Breast Cancer: What to Believe

"We are drowning in information and starving for knowledge."
ROGER RUTHERFORD

IN 1998, THERE were an estimated 178,700 new cases of female breast cancer in the United States. Over 40,000 deaths were attributed to breast cancer in 1998. As women age, their risk of breast cancer increases. Certain factors can also predispose women to developing breast cancer and include the following:

• a family history of breast cancer
• early onset of menstruation
• late menopause
• the recent use of postmenopausal estrogens
• the use of birth control pills
• breast tissue abnormalities
• giving birth at a later age
• infertility or inability to have children

In addition, the following factors may also be related to an increased risk of breast cancer:

- obesity
- lack of exercise
- a high-fat diet
- alcohol use
- exposure to pesticides or other chemicals
- induced abortion

The older a woman is when she first becomes pregnant, the higher is her risk of developing breast cancer. A woman who bears her first child after the age of thirty-five has a three times greater risk of developing breast cancer than one who delivers her first child prior to the age of eighteen. Moreover, women who never become pregnant or who never menstruate have up to a four times higher risk of developing estrogen-stimulated cancers. In addition, if a woman had an abortion—whether natural or induced—during the first trimester of her first pregnancy, she is approximately 2.5 times more likely to develop breast cancer.

Women are less at risk for developing breast cancer if they enter menopause early or their ovaries have been surgically removed. This type of hysterectomy will initiate the onset of premature menopause and is usually treated post-surgically with synthetic estrogen replacement.

What needs to be stressed here is that the most significant component that determines breast cancer risk is estrogen. Since soybeans are full of plant estrogens and estrogen promotes breast cancer, how do soybeans prevent breast cancer? It's one of nature's most fascinating paradoxes—soybeans seem to mimic the body's estrogen without having its detrimental effects.

Breast Cancer Protection and Soy: Translating the Data

The majority of studies that have looked at soy consumption for breast cancer have concluded that it appears to have a protective effect against hormonally linked cancers, but because so many factors are at play, test results need to be carefully interpreted. For example, a Chinese study of 200 women with breast cancer and 420 matched controls found that the risk for developing breast cancer was only lower in premenopausal women who ate plenty of soy. On the other hand, in a recent case-controlled trial conducted at the University of Southern California at Los Angeles, researchers interviewed 597 Asian-Americans who had already had breast cancer and found that their risk of breast cancer decreased with increasing frequency of tofu consumption in both pre- and postmenopausal women. So what do we believe? Which research gives the best answers?

If you look at studies that support the idea that soy protects breast tissue from cancer, their test results are overwhelmingly positive. They break down into epidemiological studies, laboratory test animal trials and in-vitro studies that are performed on cell cultures. Unfortunately, we are still waiting for data that would support the ability of soy to reduce breast cancer in women considered to be at high risk.

Almost 75 percent of studies conducted before 1995 show that genistein can decrease tumors in both size and number as well as protect animal subjects from exposure to carcinogenic substances. Many of these studies involved using certain chemicals that prompted the growth of breast tumors in rats. The general consensus of many of these tests is that the earlier genistein was administered, the more significant the protection. In fact, one test even suggested that soy ingestion by parents before conception ever occurred might provide a possible protective effect for future offspring. If we believe these findings, then what's the problem?

Soy's Effect on Breast Tissue: The Controversy

In the last three years, a few studies have reported that soy may stimulate the growth of certain estrogen-dependent breast cells. This news has created some confusion and concern among women. One such study conducted at the Department of Epidemiology and Biostatistics at the University of California in San Francisco found that taking thirty-eight grams of soy protein daily actually stimulated breast secretions. This particular study indicated that soy protein containing forty-five milligrams of isoflavones acted as an estrogen stimulus. While this may appear alarming, this same phenomenon occurs during pregnancy and lactation, both of which are linked to a lower risk of breast cancer. Also keep in mind that often tests conducted in vitro (test tube) will produce different results than those administered in vivo (to live subjects).

The concentrations of genistein used in these tests are also a determining factor. Some studies have found that high concentrations of genistein appear to block breast cancer cell growth in the test tube while stimulating growth in live subjects. On the other hand, dozens of other studies show that genistein is overwhelmingly protective. In fact, one 1998 study conducted on postmenopausal monkeys found that adding soy protein isolate to ERT may protect against the tumor-promoting effects of estrogen in both uterine and breast tissues. Are you even more confused now? Thirty-eight milligrams of genistein alone, which some studies used, is also higher than the amount consumed by most Asian women on a day-to-day basis.

While it is true that we lack sufficient data to evaluate the effect of soy isoflavones on normal human breast tissue, we still have enough information to make wise decisions on our soy intake. The best way to approach existing test results is to assume that taking an abnormally high dose of genistein, as part of soy protein isolate or in supplement form, may be counterproductive. On the other hand, eating very little or no soy has also been associated with negative effects. Consuming soy in moderation can do nothing but help protect our bodies and our health.

Now, we're sure many of you are scratching your head. Even well qualified scientists and physicians can have diametrically opposing views on this issue. It brings to mind Robert Mueller's comment that "Those who think they know it all are very annoying to those of us who do." While all studies must be considered to determine the optimal amount of soy isoflavones to consume and whether to take isoflavone supplements, the sheer amount of data that supports the "antiestrogen" and anticancer effect of soy isoflavones still tips the scale in soy's favor. Moreover, the overwhelming evidence in Asian cultures that soy modulates estrogen cannot be denied. The majority of all epidemiological studies that have specifically looked at soy consumption and the future incidence of breast cancer have shown that soy intake can be protective.

Common sense and prudent evaluation are needed to come to a sound conclusion concerning soy consumption. Consequently, our best bet is to look at the very effective results of soy consumption in Asian populations and assume that their statistics reflect the most beneficial and safe use of soy for breast cancer protection. To avoid soy consumption altogether because some researchers disagree, or because they haven't come to a final conclusion, could jeopardize your health. Moderate soy consumption can only benefit your body.

The National Cancer Institute and Soy

In fact, a 1990 National Cancer Institute (NCI) workshop singled out five chemical classifications of what were considered anticarcinogenic compounds in soybeans, designated as phytosterols, phytates, saponins, protease inhibitors and isoflavones. It was also noted that soybeans are rich in phenolic acids, which have anticancer properties as well. While all of these compounds are thought to contribute to the value of soy as a cancer-fighting food, it is the isoflavones that have sparked the interest of cancer researchers. The two main soybean isoflavones that have been the primary subject of study are genistein and daidzein.

On June 27, 1990, an NCI symposium held on the anticancer effects of soybeans drew the conclusion that soy foods played a profound role in the prevention of cancer. Consequently, the NCI allocated $3 million for additional research on soy foods and their ability to protect the body against cancer.

Women with Active Breast Cancer

Although soy isoflavones can clearly exert a protective effect in the prevention of breast cancer, researchers are hesitant to recommend using them for the treatment of active cancer. While some data suggests that they may actually help to inhibit the growth of active tumors, test results are still considered inconclusive. As a result, caution is the byword. Charles Simone, M.D., author of *Breast Health*, tells his patients with breast cancer to avoid soy foods because their effect on active malignancies still remains unknown. On the other hand, other doctors openly encourage their breast cancer patients to eat whole soy foods but to stay away from isoflavone supplements.

Dr. Herman Adlercreutz, a physician at Finland's University of Helsinki and a soy expert, emphasizes that there is no evidence suggesting that the amount of phytoestrogens found in foods could stimulate already existing cancer or initiate cancer growth. He also points out that eating whole soy foods, which provide the body with lignans and other anticarcinogenic compounds, makes for the complete anticancer effect. It is the diversity of all compounds found in soy that produce its desirable effects. Anytime we artificially modify or isolate these compounds, we don't know what may happen. As a result, clinicians are cautious about recommending isoflavone supplements for the treatment of active cancer. We concur and want to stress that we strongly believe in the value of some soy food as part of an overall anticancer strategy. The value of soy foods for cancer will be discussed in more detail in a later chapter. Inevitably, more research exploring whether or not soy can help to treat cancer will emerge in the near future. As it stands now, there is no data supporting the notion that soy isoflavones can either cause or cure breast cancer.

Soy Isoflavones and Breast Cancer Survivors

If you have had breast cancer or have estrogen-dependent benign breast tumors, the issue of soy consumption again sparks a great deal of controversy. Will soy act as an antiestrogen or exert an estrogenic effect on your breast tissue? This dilemma is a significant one, especially for postmenopausal women with low levels of estrogen. Will isoflavone ingestion stimulate estrogen-sensitive tumor growth? While no one can conclusively answer that question, and while some doctors may recommend that postmenopausal women stay away from soy, we believe that the amount and type of soy used make all the difference. Moderation in all things is the key. If you have had breast cancer or other breast tumors, you may want to avoid isoflavone supplements; however, the consumption of soy foods in moderate amounts and in combination with a good cancer-protective diet and healthy lifestyle would seem to be appropriate. The facts overwhelmingly support soy's protective effects. Whether or not to use drugs like Tamoxifen or other estrogen blockers to prevent a future recurrence of breast cancer is something that you should discuss with your doctor and carefully consider.

Tamoxifen Concerns

Tamoxifen was chemically engineered in the late 1960s. This drug is considered a synthetic, nonsteroidal compound with a chemical structure similar to diethylstilbestrol (DES) and shares some of the same properties. Some experts fear that it will experience the same fate as DES as its use continues over the next two decades. Tamoxifen works by preventing estrogen from binding to receptor sites on breast tissue cells much as natural phytoestrogens like soy isoflavones do. Simply stated, Tamoxifen competes with estrogen in breast tissue, thereby lessening the potential danger of estrogen binding. While Tamoxifen's effect as an antiestrogen on breast tissue seems positive enough, it exerts an estrogenic effect on the uterus and liver as well, possibly increasing the risk of endometrial and liver cancer, blood clots and other problems.

Approximately one million women with breast cancer are taking Tamoxifen. Currently, Tamoxifen is recommended for all pre-menopausal women with hormone-dependent cancers, as well as for most postmenopausal women with breast cancer. It is the most popular drug used by women with breast cancer; in fact, it is now the most widely prescribed cancer medication in the world.

In his book, *The Breast Cancer Prevention Diet,* Dr. Bob Arnot points out that while Tamoxifen can help to prevent breast cancer, it can also double the rate of uterine cancer in women over fifty. Tamoxifen clearly exerts an antiestrogenic effect, which is desirable for women who have had breast cancer, but comes, however, with a gynecological price tag. Long term use of this drug may cause serious gynecological abnormalities. Also, giving low doses of Tamoxifen to women with a high risk of breast cancer has been a controversial practice due to its potentially serious side effects.

A report published in a 1992 issue of *Lancet* contained a fascinating review of several studies involving 30,000 breast cancer patients who were randomly tagged to receive Tamoxifen or not. The patients were followed for up to six years. Of those taking Tamoxifen, 74.4 percent survived, as compared with 70.9 percent in the non-Tamoxifen group—a difference that many physicians didn't find particularly impressive. Also, there were issues of drug resistance and rebound effects, especially if the drug was taken for longer than five years.

No one really knows the risks involved in taking Tamoxifen over a long period of time. The list of potential side effects from taking Tamoxifen in the short run, however, is considerable. They include premature menopause, vaginal atrophy, fluid retention, osteoporosis, eye damage and blood clots. One study in possession of the FDA's Oncological Drugs Advisory Committee and conducted by the National Surgical Adjuvant Breast and Bowel Project in 1991 reported that the risk of developing potentially fatal blood clots is raised approximately seven fold in women taking Tamoxifen. Some Australian scientists have gone on record saying that even in small amounts, Tamoxifen has carcinogenic effects. It is, in fact, listed by the World Health Organization as a human carcinogen.

So does Tamoxifen's ability to prevent breast cancer outweigh its foibles? A study published in a 1992 issue of the *New England Journal of Medicine* reported that Tamoxifen may reduce the incidence of contralateral breast cancer, but this was demonstrated only in premenopausal women and only in three out of eight trials. Another study reported in *Octa Oncologica* found that Tamoxifen not only failed to reduce contralateral breast cancer in premenopausal women, but it actually increased incidence of this cancer. As far as postmenopausal women go, the jury is still out. Your doctor may feel that the benefits outweigh the risks; however, as far as heart disease and osteoporosis go, the positive effect of Tamoxifen is dubious. Overall, clinical trials have failed to establish that it significantly increases bone density or prevents postmenopausal heart attacks.

Soy vs. Tamoxifen

Some experts believe that due to Tamoxifen's controversy as a breast cancer preventative, using soy protein that contains isoflavones may be preferable to using the drug. In other words, taking soy may be just as effective and infinitely safer for women who are at a high risk of developing breast cancer. In his book, *What Doctors May Not Tell You about Menopause*, Dr. John Lee states: "Herbs and food contain phytoestrogens. Their benefit parallels that of Tamoxifen (without the adverse side effects) in that phytoestrogens occupy estrogen receptors and are less estrogenic than those made by the body. Since it is now known that reducing caloric intake reduces estrogen levels, and recent studies find 46 percent less breast cancer among women consuming more fruit and vegetables, it would seem that women interested in preventing breast cancer could make modest changes in diet and derive better and certainly safer results."

Regarding the potential of soy as a replacement for the drug, some studies report that soy protein containing isoflavones has anticancer actions in animal models of breast cancer and should be considered as an alternative treatment to Tamoxifen for breast cancer protection. Mark J. Messina, Ph.D. of the North Central Soybean Projects in Port Townshend, Washington, for example, believes in the safety of soy and its possible use as a Tamoxifen substitute. Other doctors and scientists are not so confident.

Our view concerning the use of soy in place of Tamoxifen has evolved from distilling existing facts among unknown variables. First of all, there are no guarantees either way that soy can replace Tamoxifen. A lack of long term studies keeps us all in the dark. We do believe, however, that soy isoflavones have the ability to protect breast tissue and that they are infinitely safer than powerful synthetic drugs even in a worst-case scenario.

TAMOXIFEN FOR HEALTHY WOMEN: ON THE WRONG TRACK?

The National Cancer Institute (NCI) decided that healthy women who are at a higher risk of getting breast cancer could benefit from Tamoxifen therapy. In April of 1992, the NCI initiated a $60 million breast cancer prevention trial that was designed to involve 16,000 healthy women in the United States, Europe, Canada and Australia. The study is still in process and is focusing on thousands of healthy women over 35 who are designated as high risk. For five years, half the women receive Tamoxifen and half take a placebo substance.

Several respected health care professionals have expressed their concern about the drug. The idea of using a potent, synthetic chemical to prevent a possible cancer is innately flawed and illustrates our unwillingness to fully address the very profound impact that dietary manipulation rather than chemical warfare can have on the incidence of cancer. Ironically, the same physicians who may warn you that soy isoflavones have not been adequately studied and may be harmful will readily fill out a prescription for drugs like Tamoxifen.

How much soy food you should consume for maximum protection still sparks debate. Some experts recommend a minimum of one serving of soy weekly while others suggest daily consumption of a soy food like tofu. It would seem that if Asian women enjoy substantial protection, imitating their dietary habits would be our best bet. Because the use of isolated soy isoflavone supplements for women with breast cancer poses some concerns, we suggest using whole soy foods instead. Soy foods act naturally with the body rather than against it.

When it comes to using soy in combination with Tamoxifen therapy, a new study suggests that genistein has a synergistic effect with the drug. According to a clinical study out of the Indiana University School of Medicine and published in the May/June 1999 issue of *AntiCancer Research,* using genistein with Tamoxifen resulted in better cancer cell inhibition, suggesting that using Tamoxifen with genistein may be of potential value in the treatment of breast cancer.

Clearly, when it comes to managing this disease, there are no easy solutions to either the prevention or treatment of breast cancer, but common sense tells us that learning to include certain foods in our diet may give us powerful protection against estrogen exposure.

Soy Fiber: Reducing Estrogen Exposure

The fiber content of soy food amounts to around six grams of fiber per one cup of cooked soybeans. The fiber-rich hull of the soybean offers the colon a number of beneficial effects. While most of us may connect the value of a high-fiber diet with colon health, few of us know that a high-fiber diet can play a profound role in breast cancer prevention as well. Several studies have looked into the role of fiber-rich foods in preventing breast cancer, and twelve case-control studies found a significant decrease in breast cancer risk in women who ate the highest amount of dietary fiber. These studies also found that women who ate the lowest quantity of cereals, beta-carotene, fruits, and vegetables had the greatest risk of developing breast cancer—keep in mind that the average American woman eats around ten grams of fiber each day. The suggested daily intake is around thirty to thirty-five grams of fiber.

A 1996 study out of the Oncology Department of St. Thomas Hospital in London reported that case-control studies in various populations around the world have concluded that a lower risk of breast cancer is linked with a higher intake of dietary fiber and complex carbohydrates. The study reported, "Although this finding has not been confirmed through American studies, the scope of its observations strongly support the notion that increasing the consumption of fiber or the use of dietary fiber supplements might reduce breast cancer risk in high-incidence populations."

Phytoestrogens and the Colon Connection

Colonic fermentation of dietary fiber actually results in the production of volatile fatty acids that may stimulate reactions and cause cancer cells to program themselves to die. Consuming phytoestrogens in the form of soy also adds a high fiber component. Since fiber works to prevent estrogen-stimulated cancers, among countless other things, the fiber content of soy works together with phytoestrogens for added benefits:

- A high-fiber diet reduces circulating estrogen by reducing the enterohepatic (from the gut through the liver) recirculation of estrogen.

- Most vegetables, including soy, contain isoflavones and lignans, which can be converted into weak estrogens in the bowel and which compete with estradiol (bad estrogen) for specific binding sites. Soy foods are particularly rich in these isoflavones.

- A high-fiber diet helps prevent obesity, which can increase availability of the biologically active 16-alpha metabolites of estrone.

• Diets rich in fiber and complex carbohydrates have been shown to improve insulin sensitivity while reducing circulating estrogen, suggesting a link between these two effects.

In other words, eating fiber helps to rid the body of bad estrogens that can initiate the formation of breast tumors. Eating plenty of plant fiber has been associated with low levels of several hormones including testosterone, estrone, androstenedion and free estradiol. Fiber helps control hormones gone awry, and soy fiber deals them a double whammy. Keep in mind that fiber helps decrease transit time and makes the stool heavier, thereby expediting the removal of estrogen from the body. Many women are unaware that a significant amount of estrogen is excreted in their bowel movements. These estrogens, which find their way into the intestines from the liver, must be eliminated. Because this waste can sit in the bowel for twenty-four hours or more, estrogen can be reabsorbed back into the body. Fiber can help to prevent this phenomenon. Remember that breast cells need estrogen to grow. If you decrease the amount of circulating estrogen in your body, you decrease your risk of breast cancer.

chapter 8

Endometrial, Colon and Prostate Cancers

"Discovery consists in seeing what everybody has seen
and thinking what nobody has thought."
ALBERT SZENT-GYORGYI

Soy and Endometrial Cancer

Endometrial cancer strikes close to 35,000 American women annually and is considered a possible risk factor if you use synthetic estrogens. A study published in the August 15, 1997 edition of the *American Journal of Epidemiology* reported that Hawaiian women who regularly eat a variety of soy foods (including tofu, soy milk and roasted soy nuts) have less than half the risk of developing endometrial cancer as do women who eat no soy. This is the first study to show an inverse correlation between soy consumption and the risk of developing uterine cancer. Rates of endometrial cancer are lower in Asia, where soy consumption is the highest. This study, titled "Association of Soy and Fiber Consumption with the Risk of Endometrial Cancer," reported that women who ate the highest amounts of phytoestrogen-rich foods, such as tofu and other soy products, had a 50 percent reduction in endometrial cancer risk, compared with those who consumed the least amounts. Dr. Marc T. Goodman, who conducted the study, concluded that diets low in calories and rich in legumes (especially soybeans), whole grain foods, vegetables and fruits reduce the risk of endometrial cancer. The study recommended that women increase consumption of soy in their diets.

Soy and Colon Cancer

Over 90,000 people are diagnosed with colon cancer annually in the United States. Colon cancer is responsible for 10 percent of all cancer deaths. In 1996, the *American Journal of Epidemiology* published a study that noted that close to 1,000 Californians who ate soybeans in some form at least once a week had half the risk of developing polyps (considered precursors to colon cancer) when compared to people who didn't eat soybeans. We've already established that soy contains five known classes of anticancer agents. The phytosterols found in soy move through the intestines to the colon and have been shown to reduce the development of colon tumors. Moreover, the saponins found in soy foods may prevent colon cancer by protecting DNA from damage and may even work to reverse the proliferation of cancerous colon cells. The complex sugars found in soy also play a protective role by boosting levels of bifidobacteria (a beneficial bacterial) in the bowel that may be associated with lower incidences of colon cancer.

To date, we have eight case-control studies on the relationship of soy and colorectal cancer in the Chinese, Japanese and in Japanese living in the United States. All of these studies found soy to be protective. More specifically, they discovered that the frequent consumption of soybeans and tofu decreased colon cancer risk. In fact, a case-controlled study involving 488 matched pairs of people, age fifty to seventy-four years old, found that a higher consumption of tofu or soybeans was inversely associated with adenomatous colorectal polyps, which are considered precursors to colorectal cancer. Consider this: those individuals who consumed one or more servings of tofu or soybeans per week had half the risk of polyps compared to those not consuming soy.

Currently, another clinical trial is underway at Michigan State University to determine if soy protein can reduce the risk of colon cancer. The study involves sixty subjects who will consume a supplement containing either thirty-eight grams of soy protein or casein (control) for one year. Results are pending.

While the exact way that soy protects us from colon cancer remains unclear, scientists believe that genistein actually reduces that amount of precancerous lesions in the colon. In fact, in an animal study, eating soy flour reduced lesions by 40 percent. Naturally, preventing colon cancer involves the same strategy prescribed for preventing all cancers: eat a diet high in plant-based, high fiber, low-fat foods, including lots of fruits and vegetables. Adding soy foods as a replacement for some animal protein only potentiates the formula.

If colon cancer runs in your family, you will be interested to know that soy protein may help reduce colon cancer incidence even in people with a history of the disease. Dr. Maurice Benninck of Michigan State University has reported to the American Institute for Cancer Research that soy intake may reduce the incidence of colon cancer by one half. Show us a prescription drug that is able to do that.

Soy for Men: Prostate Cancer Concerns

It's true that the primary thrust of this book has been to inform women about the profound value soy can offer them. It is also true that men need to acquaint themselves with the life-saving attributes of the soybean. Men typically eat too much animal protein and fatty foods, suffer from high cholesterol and are at high

WHY IS THE PROSTATE GLAND SO VULNERABLE TO DISEASE?

This walnut-sized male reproductive gland surrounds the urethra, which transports urine from the bladder to the end of the penis. The prostate gland's location explains why it enlarges and causes so many problems related to urination. The primary function of the prostate gland is to produce fluids for semen that enhance the survivability of sperm. However, due to the nature of its tissue makeup, the prostate gland is more prone to toxin accumulation—caused in part by slow blood circulation and the fatty tissue makeup of the gland. The fact that blood flow is rather sluggish in the prostate area explains why antibiotic therapy for prostatitis takes so long to clear up the infection. (Prostatitis is an inflammation of the prostate gland caused by infection, irritation or dehydration.) Prostate cancer is the second most common form of cancer in men and has prompted the American Cancer Society to recommend that men over fifty get special physical exams and blood tests to detect early cancers.

risk for prostate disease. Prostate cancer rates in America can be up to thirty times higher than the rates in some Asian cultures.

Prostate disorders are becoming increasingly common. In fact, the overwhelming consensus is that if a man lives long enough, he will inevitably face prostate problems. Currently, males between the ages of forty and sixty have a 50 percent risk factor for developing an enlarged prostate, which is a condition also referred to as benign prostatic hypertrophy (BPH). Ninety percent of men over the age of seventy suffer from BPH. To make matters worse, prostate cancer is a leading cause of death among men. Now while these statistics sound rather grim, the good news is that changing dietary habits to include soy will not only protect the prostate but will also effectively raise a man's overall health status as well.

Prostate-Protective Soy

In 1996, over 140,000 men were diagnosed with prostatic cancer, and 33,000 perished from the disease. By contrast, Asian men who eat a diet high in soy products have a low incidence of prostate cancer. Asian men who immigrate to the United States and adopt a Western diet significantly raise their risk of prostate cancer, suggesting that they have lost their soy protection. Japanese men eat between forty and seventy milligrams of genistein daily, as compared to American men who are lucky to get less than one milligram. Scientists have suspected that soy isoflavones (primarily genistein) work as chemoprotective agents in the prostate gland.

Much in the same way that soy affords breast tissue protection from estrogen, soy also prevents a certain form of testosterone and estrogen in the male body from binding to prostate receptors. Finnish clinical studies support this idea: animals given a soybean feed that consisted of 7 percent roasted soybean meal showed a significantly lower incidence of prostate tissue abnormalities when artificially stimulated with hormones. In addition, cancerous tissue that had been transplanted into test rats that ate a soy diet of 33 percent defatted soy flour developed smaller tumors than control rats on a soy-free diet. Soy worked to oppose the action of potent estrogens (DES) that prompt tumors to form in the prostate.

Another study out of the Department of Pharmacology and Toxicology at the University of Alabama at Birmingham found that soy appeared to protect against prostate cancer by inhibiting protein kinase, which can contribute to abnormal cell replication. Another fascinating study found that soy consumption was inversely related to prostate cancers in Hawaii. Dr. L. Lu and his colleagues at the University of Texas Medical Branch in Galveston looked at six men—two Indians, two African-Americans and two Caucasians—who drank about 200 milligrams of soy milk per day for one month. The study found that soy milk reduced circulating levels of dihydrotestosterone in its subjects, as well as serum levels of 17-beta-estradiol that contribute to the formation of prostate cancer.

Interestingly, some postmortem tests on elderly Asian men suggest that prostate cancer rates in Japanese men are actually the same as those found in American men; however, the Japanese cancers grow at such a slow rate that the disease often remains dormant and isn't discovered unless an autopsy is performed. The results of a new study show that mice who were inoculated with cancer cells were able to dramatically reduce the size of their tumors by eating a diet rich in soy. A team of medical researchers at Harvard Medical School has called for clinical trials to determine the effect of soy products on prostate cancer. Dr. Jin-Rong Zhou and his associates at Harvard presented their test data and stated that their results certainly warrant more investigation into soy as a treatment for prostate cancer. In addition, because cholesterol can actually accumulate in prostate tissue, using soy has additional benefits.

Dr. Electra D. Paskett, Ph.D., associate professor of public health sciences, is currently involved in a recent study of 160 men to assess the effect of soy on prostate cancer risks. The study falls under the U.S. Department of Defense's Center of Excellence in Prostate Cancer. The trial will look at 160 men, half African-American, between the ages of fifty-five and seventy who are at high risk for prostate cancer but who have normal prostate biopsies. Measurements of the effect of soybean supplements on the prostate will be taken. Unfortunately, researchers have noticed that much the same way that Asian women who come to America become more susceptible to breast cancer, Japanese men who emigrate to the United States rapidly fall into the cancer incidence rates of American men.

Soy is also a rich source of zinc, which is vitally important for the maintenance of prostate health. Zinc deficiencies have been linked to disease of the male reproductive system. Simply put, if men make a few simple changes in their diet, not only will their risk of prostate disease drop, so will their vulnerability to heart disease and cancers of all kinds drop.

Research Supports Soy's Anticancer Effect

Recently, it was reported to the American Institute for Cancer Research that instead of the previous estimate of 65 percent of experimental studies showing soy's anticancer properties, the current estimate is up to 94 percent. This jump reflects the inclusion of recent studies and was cited in the *Journal of the National Cancer Institute*. The article also mentioned that cancer researchers are anxious to get the results of a study currently underway at the University of Southern California, which involves 2,400 participants of Asian descent who live in the Los Angeles area. Dr. Anna Wu, head of this study, will be completing the study in approximately two years. Preliminary data supports the view that soy isoflavones reduce the risk of breast, prostate and endometrial cancers.

New Anticancer Gene in Soy Protein Compared to Taxol®

In addition, scientists at the University of California Berkeley have discovered a gene from soybeans that, when placed into cancer cells, produces an effect similar to the anticancer drug called Taxol®. In a recent issue of *Nature Biotechnology*, these researchers reported that this gene produces a protein called lunasin that puts a halt to the process of mitosis, which is how cells duplicate themselves. Drugs like Taxol® and Docetaxal® have potentially serious side effects, including fever, sore throat, swelling in face and hands, breathing difficulties, irregular heartbeat, numbness, nausea and hair loss. By contrast, the soy protein called lunasin not only stops cell division but also initiates certain reactions that cause the cell to eventually self-destruct without these side effects. The research team found this effect occurred in both normal and cancerous cells, including breast cancer cells.

This discovery spawns the hope that one day in the near future lunasin will be directly delivered into cancer cells (specifically those associated with ovarian and breast cancer, as well as certain types of leukemia) to prevent their replication and even cause their destruction. This would mean much safer cancer therapy without compromising effectiveness.

Soy and Other Cancers

Unquestionably, the soybean provides impressive protection for other forms of cancer. For example, a Chinese lung cancer incidence study involving over 1,200 people inversely correlated soy consumption with lung cancer rates, which went down as much as 50 percent with the addition of soy to the diet. In addition, soy milk consumption was linked with 50 percent risk reduction for stomach cancer. Test studies have also found that the Chinese have one-third the rectal cancer rates compared to test groups who ate little or not soy. In fact, a Japanese study found that soybean or tofu consumption of one to two servings per week reduced the rectal cancer risk by over 80 percent. Interestingly, the consumption of miso soup was thought to help reduce the damage caused by radiation after the bombing in Nagasaki. Soy also appears to inhibit the formation of nitrosamines, which are considered powerful carcinogens that can cause liver cancer. One study found that soy compounds worked more effectively than ascorbate to inhibit the action of nitrites found in many cured meats.

Prevention Guidelines for Any Type of Cancer

- Eat a low fat diet that is high in fiber and complex carbohydrates. Foods such as cabbage, broccoli, Brussels sprouts and cauliflower are thought by some to protect against cancer. Eat foods rich in potassium such as beans, sprouts, whole grains, almonds, sunflower seeds, sesame seeds, lentils, parsley, blueberries, coconut, endive, leaf lettuce, oats and potatoes (with the skin). Carrots and peaches are also suggested in designing an anticancer diet.

- Avoid eating fried foods, animal proteins, coffee, tea, caffeine or salt cured or smoked foods, which contain nitrites or nitrates, such as bacon, sausage, lunch meats, hot dogs and ham. In some cases, intestinal cancer may take as long as twenty years to finally develop. Some professionals recommend avoiding fluoride in water or toothpaste. Use an air purifier in your home. Do not use artificial sweeteners. (Stevia is a natural herbal sweetener that can be used.) Do not eat charred or burned foods. Never eat moldy or rancid foods.

- Don't smoke. Smoking is one of the primary causes of lung cancer that can be controlled. Smoking during pregnancy can also increase the risk of cancer to the offspring. Avoid breathing second-hand smoke as well.

- Do not drink alcohol heavily; heavy drinkers are at greater risk for mouth, throat, esophagus, stomach and liver cancers.

- Some studies have shown that germanium may be a factor in the prevention of cancer.

- Take a good strong antioxidant array supplement every day.

- Women should take cruciferous indole supplements if they are at high risk for breast cancer; they should also eat a daily serving of soy.

- If cancer runs in your family, get an annual checkup and watch for any warning signs of the disease.

- In some countries where breast cancer is low, iodine content in soils is particularly high; therefore, an iodine deficiency may be linked to the incidence of breast cancer. Likewise, areas low in selenium have also been linked to a higher rate of cancer. Make sure you're getting enough iodine and selenium.

• Obesity has been linked to certain types of cancer, such as uterine or breast cancer. Stay at an optimum weight for your height and frame.

• Some studies have linked a higher incidence of prostate cancer for males to those who have had a vasectomy.

• Men should take saw palmetto and pygeum supplements after the age of forty to prevent prostate cancer.

• Avoid unnecessary x-rays.

• Avoid exposure to chemicals such as paint, garden pesticides, (which are considered high-risk carcinogens), hair sprays and sunlight. Get in the habit of using a strong sunscreen. Avoid exposure to asbestos, vinyl chloride, industrial dyes and soot.

• Have your home checked for radon gas levels.

• Take screening tests for early detection of breast, cervical, colon and intestinal cancer.

• Exercise regularly. Exercise increases the efficiency of the immune system.

• Practice safe sex. Venereal disease has been linked to the development of cervical cancer, not to mention the danger of AIDS, which can itself lead to the contraction of cancer.

chapter 9

Bone Health
and Osteoporosis
Prevention

"If I'd known I was gonna live this long, I'd have taken better care of myself."
EUBIE BLAKE, AT AGE 100

TWENTY MILLION WOMEN in the United States suffer from osteoporosis. This debilitating condition is considered a major health problem. In 1990, more than 1.5 million bone fractures were reported worldwide that were attributed to osteoporosis. The majority of these fractures occurred in women, who comprise the greatest risk group for the disease. As a woman ages, her chances of suffering a bone fracture dramatically increase. One out of every five American women will fracture one or more bones from the age of sixty-five onward.

Osteoporosis is nothing more than a reduction in bone tissue, resulting in the creation of brittle and fragile bones that are susceptible to fracture. The disease typically strikes postmenopausal women and older men and has been attributed to hormonal changes (such as a decline of estrogen and progesterone) and a lack of calcium or vitamin D. In women, estrogen promotes bone formation and density, which keeps bones fracture-resistant.

Consider the fact that in the first three to five years after menopause, women lose an average of 3–5 percent of their bone mass annually. This loss will eventually taper off but will increase again after the age of eighty. As is the case with so many of the conditions we've discussed, osteoporosis is directly linked with Western eating habits and lifestyles. For example, a study reported in a 1993 edition of *Epidemiology* stated that the more caffeine you consume, the greater your bone loss will be. We have found that the following factors contribute to the development of osteoporosis:

- excess animal protein and sodium consumption
- caffeine consumption
- lack of calcium in the diet
- removal of the ovaries
- Cushing's syndrome
- lack of mobility
- lack of sunshine or vitamin D
- prolonged use of corticosteroid drugs
- tobacco and alcohol consumption
- malabsorption of nutrients from food
- genetic predisposition
- using blood thinners, some anticonvulsants and synthroid (l-thyroxine or thyroid hormone)

In addition, we have also found that the following conditions often predisposed our patients to the disease:

- never having been pregnant
- having a fragile frame and fair skin
- being underweight
- consuming too much iron
- presence of digestive disorders
- early menopause
- diabetes
- chronic pulmonary disease
- rheumatoid arthritis

Note: Osteoporosis is also a problem for men. A 1995 study published in the *British Journal of Rheumatology* revealed that 30 percent of all hip fractures occur in men and that vertebral fractures are much more common in men than previously thought. The female-to-male ratio is only 2 to 1. The study stressed that men in their sixties are not adequately warned that as their testosterone levels decline, their bones may become weaker. Male menopause, or andropause, is a factor to be considered. Men, like women, could benefit from taking supplemental calcium and vitamin D, as well as consuming at least one serving of soy per day.

The Calcium Controversy

Consider the fact that Asian and vegetarian women have a lower incidence of osteoporosis than Western women, who ingest similar or even higher amounts of calcium. Obviously, calcium consumption alone is not enough. It doesn't matter how much calcium you consume if you end up losing most of it because of poor absorption. In fact, eating animal protein (instead of soy protein) has a detrimental effect on how calcium is absorbed and utilized. These proteins cause calcium to be excreted in the urine, and the more calcium you lose, the less is available to maintain bone density. According to a study published in the *American Journal of Clinical Nutrition,* women who were vegetarians for at least twenty years have an average bone mineral loss of 18 percent by the time they turn eighty, compared to a 35 percent loss for those who have been meat eaters. Not all protein causes this effect—soy protein causes less excretion of calcium than animal protein.

For example, in one study, test subjects consumed all of their protein in the form of animal products, such as beef, fish and chicken, and they excreted approximately 150 milligrams of calcium per day. By contrast, when all of their protein came from a soy source, they excreted only 103 milligrams of calcium. A difference of forty-seven milligrams per day could significantly impact bone density over a long period of time. The ability to conserve calcium is vitally important for both men and women.

Bones experience a continuous state of regeneration. Seven thousand milligrams of calcium enter and exit bones every day, and the kind of protein found in soy enhances calcium retention. On the other hand, eating foods like meat, eggs, etc., can deplete our calcium reserves. In fact, scientists have found that for every one gram increase in animal protein consumption, an average loss of 1.75 milligrams of calcium will occur. Animal protein foods contain sulfur amino acids, cysteine and methionine, which are believed to elevate acids that lead to calcium loss.

Considering the over-consumption of animal protein, which we commonly see in the United States, it's no wonder that osteoporosis affects so many women. Moreover, many women are unaware that many soy foods can provide them with rich sources of bioavailable calcium. Conventional medicine offers relatively new treatments for osteoporosis—including drugs such as Alendronate, Calcitonin and Raloxifene, which are often given with calcium supplementation—but these drugs also come with significant side effects.

Soy Foods as Sources of Calcium

Despite common beliefs, dairy products are not the only viable source of calcium. Women in other countries who consume scarce amounts of dairy foods get their calcium in ample supply from plant sources. Soy foods are an excellent source of calcium. Tofu, fortified soy milk, tempeh, soybeans and textured vegetable protein are all considered good dietary sources of calcium. For example, one cup of cooked soybeans contains 175 milligrams of calcium, and one serving of tofu can provide 120 to 750 milligrams of calcium. In addition, soy milk that has been fortified with calcium is an excellent source, providing nearly 30 percent of the adult RDA per one-cup serving.

Osteoporosis is more common in people with lactose intolerance because they avoid milk products. Some vegetables are also good sources of calcium but contain oxalic acid and other compounds that may inhibit calcium absorption by as much as 60 percent. Some of these calcium-rich vegetables are broccoli, kale, spinach and turnip, mustard and collard greens. Other foods high in oxalic acid are beet greens, almonds, cashews, chard and rhubarb. Foods that can decrease calcium absorption include cocoa, bran and wheat germ. High fiber drinks and supplements can also interfere with calcium assimilation. Researchers say, however, that these substances seem to interfere with calcium absorption only when calcium intake is low. Supplementation of vitamin D and magnesium also can help with calcium absorption.

The Vitamin K Connection

Dr. Kironobu Katsuyama and his associates at the Kawasaki Medical School in Japan conducted a study on natto, a fermented soybean product that contains high levels of vitamin K, which they believe plays an important role in the formation of bone. They referred to previous studies that reported that people who ate natto were less likely to suffer from hip fractures in old age— a very common occurrence in people with osteoporosis. Natto has one hundred times as much of a specific type of vitamin K (K2) as cheese does. The study looked at local workers who consumed natto. Dr. Katsuyama tested these people for a known genetic deficiency that inhibits the body's ability to absorb calcium. People with this impaired gene do not absorb vitamin D properly, which is vital for calcium assimilation. Vitamin D is actually produced in the skin when it is exposed to sunlight.

The study discovered that people with this genetic problem who did not eat natto suffered from calcium loss. Those people, however, who had the faulty gene and ate natto retained calcium and, as a result, maintained durable bone mass. Dr. Katsuyama's team concluded that the vitamin K2 content of natto must participate in calcium retention. They are pursuing more follow-up studies. Phytonutrients found in foods work in ways we may not recognize or understand to promote health. This notion builds the case for eating foods in their whole state as nature intended.

Soy's Impact on Bone: Clinical Findings

The ability of soy isoflavones to increase bone mineral density in postmenopausal women has been noted in both animal and human studies. Several animal studies performed on rats that had their ovaries removed found that both genistein and daidzein inhibited bone breakdown. One such study, published in the January 1999 issue of the *Journal of Nutrition,* was conducted at the Chicago campus of the University of Illinois in Urbana. In September 1999, researchers there found that soy isoflavones could help to fortify the bones found in the lumbar spine and also help to prevent the dowager's hump commonly seen in postmenopausal women suffering from osteoporosis. This study involved sixty-six postmenopausal women who consumed forty grams of isolated soy protein daily containing either fifty-six milligrams or ninety milligrams of mixed isoflavones for a period of twenty-four weeks. Only those women consuming the higher level of isoflavones had a significant increase in bone mineral density and bone mineral content in the lumbar spine. The authors noted that the spine, compared to the other measured skeletal sites, is considered the most sensitive to estrogen, due to its high content of trabecular bone—which can change more rapidly than other bone locations. In an Australian trial of fifty-two postmenopausal women, those patients who consumed forty-five grams of soy grits per day for a twelve-week period also experienced a significant increase in bone mineral content in the spine.

As we mentioned earlier, most women lose 2–3 percent of their bone density in the initial two to three years following menopause, suggesting that the sooner isoflavone consumption is increased, the better. One of the primary reasons women may choose to take estrogen replacement therapy (ERT) after menopause is to protect their bone density. However, one study discovered that using genistein resulted in the retention of bone mineral mass equivalent to prescription doses of estradiol. Genistein may also positively affect other enzymes in bone cells that work to maintain the integrity of the bone. By so doing, the bone-thinning process that occurs after menopause may be minimized.

Another way that genistein may help preserve bone health is by inhibiting the action of osteoclasts, which are cells that work to remove bone tissue. Some studies have also reported that treatment with genistein decreased the loss of bone mineral density and volume, suggesting that genistein may actually stimulate the formation of bone—something that prescription estrogen drugs can't do. Dr. Paolo Fanti of the University of Kentucky in Lexington has pointed out that the protective effect of synthetic estrogen on bone works through a suppression of bone tissue turnover. By contrast, genistein enhances bone production while reducing bone loss.

Soy Protein as a Treatment for Active Osteoporosis

In another report, Dr. Bahram Arjmandi, a soy researcher at the Department of Human Nutrition and Dietetics at the University of Illinois at Chicago, found that soy protein may be a natural alternative therapy for women who already suffer from osteoporosis. His clinical trial examined whether soy protein isolate would prevent or slow bone loss. The study, reported in a 1998 issue of the *American Journal of Clinical Nutrition*, found that while bone density increased with the consumption of soy isolate, more importantly, bone quality improved. Dr. Arjmandi has stressed the profound implications of using soy for the ever-increasing number of Americans who suffer from the disease.

Soy's Boron Boost

Soybeans are a rich source of boron, a mineral that may help to prevent osteoporosis. It is thought that boron may actually stimulate endogenous estradiol 17B in and of itself by acting like a mild form of ERT. Moreover, boron is required for bone mineralization. If you lack boron, your bones cannot maintain the critical levels of calcium they require for good bone integrity. In a study conducted by Dr. Forrest H. Nielsen at the USDA Human Nutrition Research Center in North Dakota, postmenopausal women consuming low-boron diets more easily lost calcium and magnesium. By adding three milligrams of boron to their diet, their calcium losses dropped by 40 percent. Eating soy foods can help supply the body with boron.

Genistein vs. Premarin for Osteoporosis Prevention

According to Dr. J. Anderson and his research team at the Department of Nutrition and Dental Research at the University of North Carolina at Chapel Hill, a low dose of genistein had an effect similar to that of Premarin in maintaining bone tissue. At higher doses, however, genistein did not. Both Premarin and genistein suppress production of cytokine, which is involved in bone loss and regeneration. Dr. Anderson published a review entitled "The Effects of Phytoestrogens on Bone" in a 1995 issue of the *Journal of Nutrition Research* in which he discussed experimental studies of the effect of soy (isoflavones) on bone density. After investigating human, animal and test tube trials, he concluded that soy isoflavones (especially genistein and daidzein), if taken in proper doses, could improve bone mass. In fact, researchers noted that certain levels of genistein are as effective as the powerful prescription estrogen replacement drug Premarin. It has also been pointed out in various medical journals that the way synthetic estrogen is administered influences its impact on bone. Some studies even claim that osteoporosis actually begins in the years prior to menopause when estrogen levels are still high. This suggests another possible causal component—low progesterone levels.

Interestingly, optimal doses of genistein were not large. In fact, comparatively speaking, smaller doses seem more effective or equal to larger doses when it comes to the percent of bone mineral retention. Remember that total isoflavone content needs to be broken down into genistein and daidzein amounts. Ongoing studies are in process to further evaluate the effect of soy on bone integrity.

Ipriflavone: Potentiated Isoflavone Compound for Bone Health

In 1988, the Japanese registered an osteoporosis drug called Ipriflavone, which is nothing more that a synthetic isoflavone compound with daidzein as one of its metabolites. Ipriflavone has been used in Europe and Japan to treat bone loss and is now available as a dietary supplement. Ipriflavone has the distinct ability to increase the activity of bone-building cells, called osteoblasts, while inhibiting the action of osteoclasts, which actually break down bone material. One study conducted in 1998 found that Ipriflavone was able to dramatically boost new bone formation and repair. Fifty-six postmenopausal women with low bone density all received 1,000 milligrams of calcium, and random subjects were given an additional 600 milligrams of Ipriflavone. The women who only took the calcium actually experienced increased bone loss after two years. By contrast, bone loss was totally halted in those who took the Ipriflavone. The study concluded, "Ipriflavone prevents the rapid bone loss following early menopause." Ipriflavone does not have estrogenic actions in and of itself. It does, however, boost estrogen action in the body.

The recommended dosage of Ipriflavone is 600 milligrams daily. It must be stressed here, however, that even in the midst of favorable data, Ipriflavone is still considered a synthetic and artificially potentiated isoflavone—no data exists that examines any possible negative effects from its long-term use. Carl Germano, R.D, William Cabot, M.D., and Lisa Turner, authors of *The Osteoporosis Solution*, recommend taking 600 milligrams (200 milligrams three times daily) of Ipriflavone with 1,000 milligrams of calcium (in the citrate form) for osteoporosis prevention. Since Ipriflavone is a synthetically formulated compound, however, it is not accepted by the body in the same ways as whole soy foods are. Your decision to use Ipriflavone should be based on your predisposition to osteoporosis and other alternative measures you can take.

Guidelines for Osteoporosis Prevention

Women who are approaching menopause and are at risk for developing osteoporosis should consult their physician about a bone density study to evaluate their skeletal status. Some doctors dispute the value of this type of diagnosis. Discuss its advantages with your doctor. However, consider getting a bone evaluation, because although osteoporosis can begin at menopause, it can also be symptomless for a long period of time. Often the first sign of the disease is discovered when a minor fall causes a fracture. Typical sites for these fractures are above the wrist and the top of the femur. Fractures of one or several vertebrae can also occur and result in a progressive loss of height and a curvature of the spine. In these cases, compression of the spinal cord may cause chronic back pain.

Calcium and Vitamin D

In general, adult women should make sure they get enough calcium and vitamin D for protection against osteoporosis. In August 1997, the Institute of Medicine of the National Academy of Sciences issued a report stating that both men and women ages nineteen to fifty should consume 1,000 milligrams of calci-

THE EXERCISE COMPONENT

When it comes to fighting osteoporosis, the importance of weight exercises cannot be overemphasized. Increasing bone density early in life is particularly important in preventing osteoporosis. Exercise helps to build bone and maintain its mass. Even if calcium is present in the body, without exercise the bones will not take it up. Studies indicate that a sufficient amount of exercise can maintain bone strength at abnormally high levels for an indefinite period of time. Use weights, equipment or exercises that provide resistance.

um per day, and those over fifty years should consume 1,200 milligrams per day. A recent study reports that calcium citrate supplementation (400 milligrams, twice daily) prevents bone loss and stabilizes bone density in early postmenopausal women. A randomized, placebo-controlled study conducted at the Center for Mineral Metabolism and Clinical Research at the University of Texas Southwestern Medical Center reported that calcium citrate appears to inhibit bone loss and has superior bone-sparing properties. Its high bioavailability in the body is thought to be a factor. Apparently, when calcium citrate is given on an empty stomach, it is better absorbed than calcium carbonate. Make sure to take vitamin D with your calcium.

Some people have questioned whether calcium and soy can be taken together. Although soy contains substances such as phytate and oxalate that bind certain minerals such as calcium, bioavailability data on calcium indicate that absorption from tofu and soy is similar to that from milk. Also, soy is relatively high in calcium. Recommended sources of calcium are soy foods like soy milk, tofu, buttermilk, buckwheat, kelp, founder, nuts, oats, cheese, whole wheat, yogurt, skim milk, and sardines.

Magnesium, Boron, Copper and Zinc

Use a magnesium supplement to ensure proper calcium assimilation, and take 500 milligrams daily. Boron and copper are two minerals that also improve the uptake of calcium and make up certain compounds in the bone. Soy is a significant source of boron, and zinc may be the perfect complement to soy isoflavones. A study published in 1998 reports that zinc, an essential trace element, has also been shown to enhance bone formation and inhibit bone reabsorption, both in live and test tube trials. This study looked at the relationship between genistein and zinc and the effects of this combination on bone metabolism of elderly female rats. These researchers found that the isoflavonoid effect was enhanced by zinc. Keep in mind also that if you have a deficiency of hydrochloric acid (HCL) in your stomach, you won't absorb calcium properly.

Natural Progesterone Cream

Dr. John Lee's work suggests that a good natural progesterone cream may help to prevent or even reverse osteoporosis. In 1981, Dr. Lee conducted a landmark study that indicated it is the cessation of progesterone production in postmenopausal women that causes the development of osteoporosis. Contrary to current trends, progesterone replacement, not estrogen, may really be the answer to preventing and treating osteoporosis.

Dietary Guidelines

Along with daily servings of soy foods, eat a diet high in fruits and vegetables and low in fat and animal protein. Increase your consumption of flavonoid-rich foods, such as dark colored berries and fruits. Limit high protein animal foods, caffeine and alcohol. Avoid carbonated drinks. The phosphates contained in these beverages can cause calcium to be excreted in excess amounts. Colas and carbonated drinks in particular are often high in phosphoric acid and should be avoided. Do not smoke. Smoking accelerates bone loss in both men and women.

chapter 10

Soy for Heart Health

"Take care of your body with steadfast fidelity. The soul must see through these eyes alone, and if they are dim, the whole world is clouded."
JOHANN WOLFGANG VON GOETHE

ADDING SOY FOODS to your diet is a simple but powerful way to protect your heart. Soy foods are low in saturated fat, provide protein and are completely free of cholesterol. The contrast between the cardiovascular health of Asians as compared to Americans is compelling—among men forty-five to sixty-five years of age, the rates of coronary heart disease (CHD) deaths are about six times lower in Japan than the United States. For women, CHD rates are about eight-fold lower in Japan than in women of the same age in the United States.

Close to three million of us take prescription drugs for high cholesterol, and while these drugs can be effective, they come with significant side effects. Moreover, many of us are walking time bombs because we are totally unaware that we suffer from high cholesterol levels. Estimates are that over thirty-five million Americans have a total serum cholesterol count of over 240, which puts them at considerable risk for cardiovascular disease.

Interestingly, even if your cholesterol count falls in the range of 200–239 (as it does for over 55 million people), your risk of heart disease is double that of individuals whose cholesterol levels are below 200. High cholesterol levels can also contribute to gallstones, impotence, mental impairment and high blood pressure.

Heart-Healthy Soy: Cholesterol Buster

In 1995, the *New England Journal of Medicine* published an analysis of soy and concluded that "the consumption of soy protein rather than animal protein significantly decreased serum concentrations of total cholesterol, LDL cholesterol [the bad kind] and triglycerides without significantly affecting serum HDL cholesterol [the good kind] concentrations." (The terms "good" and "bad" cholesterol were coined by one of our authors, Dr. Neil Solomon.) Thirty-eight controlled clinical trials were included in the review. The average intake of soy protein was forty-seven grams per day, equivalent to the amount in one half cup of soy flour, and the average decrease in total cholesterol was 9.3 percent. In practical terms, this means that if your total cholesterol was 220 and you added one half cup of soy flour to your daily diet, your cholesterol level would decrease to 200. This drop in blood cholesterol levels represents a 20–30 percent reduction in heart disease risk, which is significant.

Keep in mind also that when cholesterol is artificially lowered, the good kind of cholesterol (HDL), as well as the bad kind (LDL), drops, and that's not a good thing. Soy protein lowers only the LDL cholesterol, or what we like to call "the least desirable cholesterol," without effecting HDL levels. Moreover, adding soy to your diet can also reduce the amount of cholesterol that is oxidized. Cholesterol becomes oxidized when it reacts with oxygen in the body. It is this oxidized form of cholesterol that causes damage to the artery walls. In one study, subjects who ate soy every day for six months experienced a 50 percent reduction in the amount of blood cholesterol that was oxidized compared to those who didn't eat soy. Based on this data, Dr. Takemichi Kanazaw of Hirosake University School of Medicine in Japan believes that soy can be very useful in the prevention of vascular disease.

Other Ways That Soy Protects the Cardiovascular System

Dr. Mary Astuti of Gadjah Mada University in Togyakarta, Indonesia also found that tempeh, which is produced from fermented soy, contains the antioxidant enzyme superoxide dismutase (SOD), which also prevents undesirable lipid peroxidation. Dr. Alan Chart of the University of Washington in Seattle found that genistein and daidzein may work similar to vitamin C in scavenging for free radicals in a water soluble environment (blood). These free radicals can make artery walls more susceptible to cholesterol (plaque) buildup. The beneficial effect of soy isoflavones on arteries has also been supported by Dr. Norberta Schoene of the Beltsville Human Nutrition Research Center in Beltsville, Maryland. She reported that soy isoflavones may positively affect cardiovascular disease because they appear to inhibit clot formations, which can obstruct blood vessels.

Simply stated, soy protein works in three ways to better our cholesterol profile:

• It decreases cholesterol absorption.
• It increases cholesterol excretion.
• It lowers circulating levels of LDL cholesterol.

An added bonus is that soy isoflavones also have antioxidant and anticlotting effects that help to prevent artery damage.

It's in the Isoflavones

One reason why it's so important to read labels on soy foods is that any soy product without isoflavones will not give us the cardiovascular benefits seen in clinical studies. For example, at the Bowman Gray School of Medicine, J. Koudy Williams, D.V.M., fed twenty-two monkeys diets containing soy protein with or without isoflavones. When the monkeys' hearts experienced stress through artificial stimulation, those monkeys who had eaten soy with isoflavones maintained normal heart function; those who had eaten soy without isoflavones developed heart abnormalities. In another study, soy protein that contained isoflavones caused the greatest decline in LDL cholesterol levels in laboratory animals.

Scientists have recently reported that the cholesterol-lowering effect of soy depends largely on the amount of isoflavones that is present. The higher the amount of isoflavones in the soy, the larger the beneficial effect will be. Keep in mind once again that using isolated isoflavone supplements may not result in the same effects. Researchers have found that isoflavones that have been extracted from soy do not lower cholesterol. Moreover, the cholesterol-lowering power of soy seems to be dose-dependent. For example, the more tofu you eat, the better result you should obtain. Studies have found that eating one-fourth to one-half of a cake of tofu daily yielded a significant drop in LDL cholesterol.

While most scientific focus has been on genistein, a study in progress at Wake Forest University is looking at daidzein specifically and has already found that daidzein, rather than genistein, may be of even greater cardiovascular value. The ratio between these two isoflavones is also significant and falls between three to one and four to one (genistein to daidzein). Most studies to date have focused on genistein as the active ingredient in preventing cardiovascular diseases and cancer. This new study will explore the synergistic role of the two compounds. Once again, you can see why eating soy in its natural state gives us an isoflavone ratio as designed by Mother Nature, who always seems to know what she's doing.

Soy for Children with High Cholesterol

Statistics concerning the heart health of our children are nothing less than appalling. An estimated 36 percent of American youth age nineteen, which is over twenty-seven million children, have serum cholesterol levels of 170 or higher (this is comparable to a level of 200 in adults). The American Heart Association has warned that artery disease can begin in young people. Compelling evidence exists that the atherosclerotic process begins in childhood and progresses slowly into adulthood.

Our children typically eat diets full of saturated fat and sugar and rarely eat the whole grains, fiber, fresh fruits and vegetables they need. Be mindful that if you just decrease animal protein in the diets of your children, they may still be at risk. Eating the combination of sugar and hydrogenated fats found in many baked goods and snacks can be just as bad if not worse than eating animal fats.

Soy foods offer children tremendous health benefits. Unfortunately, the soy intake of American children is practically negligible. In 1992, the American Academy of Pediatrics issued recommendations that an optimal diet for children should not contain more than 30 percent fat and a maximum of 10 percent saturated fat. Interestingly, even a reduction of saturated fat for some children with high cholesterol had less than impressive results, suggesting that a genetic component was at work. Approximately 1 percent of all children suffer from a genetic defect that predisposes them to high cholesterol levels.

Dr. K. Widhalm, of the Department of Pediatrics at the University of Vienna in Austria, found that just reducing the saturated fat intake of these children was not enough, even after three years of dietary adjustments. He conducted a study comparing the use of plant proteins with animal proteins in twenty-three children with high cholesterol counts. The plant protein diet contained approximately twenty grams of soy protein isolate, which had been mixed into usual foods. In the group consuming the soy protein, cholesterol levels went down 16–22 percent. Dr.

Widhalm pointed out that the use of cholesterol-lowering drugs should be avoided as long as possible and the use of soy protein could offer an effective way to considerably reduce the cholesterol counts of children and adolescents. Dr. Christine Williams, a pediatrician at the American Health Foundation who works with children suffering from high cholesterol levels, suggests sneaking soy protein into good-tasting tofu shakes (refer to the recipe section).

Which Kind of Soy Is Best?

In studies, soy protein consumed at a level of twenty-five grams significantly lowered LDL cholesterol—so much so in fact, that the Food and Drug Administration (FDA) has authorized a health claim for soy foods stating the relationship between soy protein and heart disease risk reduction. It is the protein component of soy that contains the isoflavones thought to be responsible for this cholesterol-lowering effect. Again, we all need to get more soy savvy and learn to look for the protein content of soy foods. Soy protein isolate, found in some beverages, bars and other products (like newly developed cereals from Kellogg's and General Mills and flour products from the widely recognized Arrowhead Mills), can also be effective. Dr. Craig Winkel of Georgetown University, author of several soy studies, believes that you can successfully lower bad cholesterol while raising good cholesterol with soy protein. Today, researchers are trying to hone in on the most effective quantities of soy to consume for optimal heart health. In the meantime, many health care experts are recommending adding two servings of soy-based food to your diet daily, which will also serve to lower your overall fat and animal protein intake.

Soy and Postmenopausal Heart Disease

One of the most serious concerns women have in deciding whether or not to go on hormone replacement therapy (HRT) is that some data suggests that without it, a women's risk of heart disease escalates. Once again, soy isoflavones seem tailor-made for this problem because they target virtually all major health concerns related to menopause, including heart disease. A Japanese study published in 1998 involving close to 5,000 test subjects reported that substantial soy consumption strongly correlated to lower cholesterol levels. Moreover, in a 1997 issue of *Fertility and Sterility*, data from a clinical study found that soy isoflavones appear to boost vascular function and protect the heart, suggesting that using soy supplements may be an alternative to HRT for women concerned about their risk of heart attack.

Dr. Sulistiyani of the Primate Research Center at Bogor Agricultural University in Indonesia believes that one of the primary reasons estrogen replacement therapy (ERT) is so effective in helping to reduce the risk of coronary heart disease in postmenopausal women is its antioxidant properties. However, we already know that HRT is associated with an increased risk of certain cancers and can cause a whole host of unwanted side effects. In addition, one of the latest studies on HRT claims that it actually increased the risk of heart disease during the first year or so of its use.

In a recent study using female monkeys who had their ovaries removed to simulate postmenopausal women, it was shown that genistein inhibited LDL oxidation by 48 percent. When used in combination with vitamin E, this effect was even better. What this suggests is that soy protein offers powerful heart-protective properties for everyone and may be especially desirable for postmenopausal women, who could also use its other estrogenic benefits.

Postmenopausal Strokes and Soy

At an American Heart Association meeting, Wake Forest University researchers reported that postmenopausal hormone replacement therapy from soy protein with phytoestrogens provides equivalent reduction in the occurrence of atherosclerosis in the internal carotid artery to the standard Premarin therapy. A blockage of this artery is considered a leading cause of stroke.

Thomas Clarkson, D.V.M., professor of comparative medicine at the Wake Forest University School of Medicine, praised the effectiveness of soy phytoestrogens. He pointed out that stroke is the third leading cause of death for middle-aged and post-menopausal women, and the value of using HRT to reduce the risk of stroke is still considered questionable. For this reason, Dr. Clarkson stressed that using soy phytoestrogens to prevent plaque deposits in the carotid artery may be the best way to lower stroke incidence in older women.

Soy Awareness and the FDA

In light of the fact that soy awareness is changing from what were previously apathetic attitudes toward soy, the FDA recently finalized the Soy Protein Health Claim, which associates soy protein with a reduced risk of coronary heart disease (CHD). Now any company producing a food or food substances under the FDA's jurisdiction can make a legitimate health claim if the product meets the guidelines of the rule.

In order to qualify, the soy food must contain at least 6.25 grams of soy protein per reference amount customarily consumed (RACC). Additional criteria state that the food must contain 3 grams or less of fat, 1 gram or less of saturated fat and 20 milligrams or less of cholesterol, and the food must meet specific sodium restrictions. Exceptions to the fat content of this rule include food products that consist of or are derived from whole soybeans and contain no additional fat to the fat naturally found in the whole soybean.

FDA-approved label statements can now read, "25 grams of soy protein a day, as part of a diet low in saturated fat and cholesterol, may reduce the risk of heart disease. A serving of (name of food) supplies xx grams of soy protein." In addition, you may also see the following approved statement: "Diets low in saturated fat and cholesterol that include 25 grams of soy protein a day may reduce the risk of heart disease. One serving of (name of food) provides xx grams of soy protein."

In light of this, it will become even more important for us as consumers to be able to recognize what soy products truly live up to their claims. Remember that all soy foods are not created equal. Deciding whether only soy foods that contain isoflavones deserve this special labeling is yet to be determined. (Incidentally, some of the new cholesterol-lowering margarines and salad dressings have used soy compounds to create their food formulas.)

Complementary Herbs for Cholesterol Control

Red Yeast Rice

Unquestionably, one of the most impressive compounds for controlling cholesterol is extracted from red yeast rice and is known as monascus went rice, or rice that has been fermented by the addition of yeast. Asians eat between fourteen and fifty-five grams of red yeast rice daily, sprinkling it on main dishes like tofu as a colorful topping, and it's no coincidence that their cholesterol levels are significantly lower than ours. Tofu coupled with red yeast rice deals heart disease a double blow. Mevinoilin, a natural compound found in red yeast rice, contains HGM-CoA inhibitors that safely block the production of cholesterol in the liver.

OTHER WAYS TO CONTROL YOUR CHOLESTEROL

To manage your cholesterol, first lower your consumption of saturated, hydrogenated and even polyunsaturated fats. Use olive oil and canola oil, and try to eat cold water fish more than once a week. Learn to exercise regularly, and if you're overweight, lose those extra pounds (for every ten pounds of fat you carry, you make 100 milligrams of cholesterol daily).

One of the best things you can do to control cholesterol is to eat more fiber. A 1999 study confirms that adding wheat fiber to your diet can protect you from heart disease by lowering blood fats; wheat fiber is also great for losing weight. Remember that cooked, whole soybeans are a rich source of fiber. If you're a fiber phobic, fiber supplements that contain psyllium and guar gum work well.

You should also limit your consumption of animal meats, dairy products, lard and related items and avoid solid margarines that contain transfatty acids. Eat plenty of whole grains, raw fruits (such as raisins, dried figs and dates) and vegetables. In addition, limit your intake of white flour and white sugar.

Scores of Chinese studies confirm the ability of red yeast rice to lower cholesterol. The most recent American study was conducted by Dr. David Heber, founder and director of the Center for Human Nutrition at the University of California at Los Angeles and a director of the American Board of Nutrition. Using placebo-controlled randomized methods, Dr. Heber studied eighty-three people with moderately high cholesterol levels. Those who just modified their diet but did not receive red yeast rice supplementation experienced no change in their cholesterol levels over a period of eight to twelve weeks. By contrast, the group who used the same diet and took red yeast rice had a marked drop in their cholesterol—from an average of 250 to 210 milligrams per deciliter over twelve weeks.

Red yeast rice is considered nontoxic; however, anyone taking prescription drugs to control cholesterol levels should not take red yeast rice without their doctor's approval. In addition, red yeast rice is not recommended for anyone with yeast allergies, liver disease or women who are pregnant or breast-feeding. Look for products that contain a standardized percentage of Mevinoilin. Customary dosages are to take 500 milligrams in the morning and 500 milligrams in the afternoon for a total of 1,000 milligrams per day.

Gugulipid

This exotic sounding herb is actually a gum extract from the mukul myrrh tree, which is native to India. It contains two bioactive compounds that work to normalize cholesterol levels. Numerous clinical studies using gugulipid support its ability to lower LDL while raising HDL. How does it work? Compounds in this herb work by stimulating the liver to increase the amount of LDL cholesterol it filters out of the bloodstream. It also stimulates the thyroid gland, which positively affects blood fat levels and is linked to weight loss as well. Gugulipid supplementation can lower total blood cholesterol, blood triglycerides and LDL (bad cholesterol) while raising blood HDL (good cholesterol). A 1994 study of 61 patients found that fifty milligrams of gugulipid taken twice daily for twenty-four weeks decreased the total cholesterol by 11.7 percent, the LDL cholesterol by 12.5 percent and triglycerides by 12.0 percent. Researchers concluded that gugulipid, in combination with a good diet, was as effective as prescription drugs in lowering cholesterol. Gugulipid can also help prevent atherosclerosis and may even work to reverse existing cholesterol deposits.

The dosage of gugulipids depends on the guggulsterone content of the product, which should be at 5 percent. Take twenty-five milligrams of guggulsterones three times daily (which translates to 500 milligrams of a 5 percent guggulsterone product per day). Gugulipid is considered nontoxic, but if you're taking drugs for your cholesterol, check with your doctor before starting any supplementation.

chapter 11

Little-Known Properties of Soy Isoflavones

"The essence of knowledge is, having it, to apply it;
not having it, to confess your ignorance."
CONFUCIUS

WE HOPE THAT by now you've gained an appreciation for soy's extraordinary nutritive profile. Let's talk about some of soy's other hallmarks that few of us know about. Be assured that manufacturers who are smart enough to keep their finger on the public pulse are currently busy designing new soy foods. Over 10,000 soy-based products can be found on store shelves. You may have already seen soy dogs, soy cheese, soy bacon, soy sausage and soy cream cheese at your local grocery store. Some of these products taste good. Others taste—well, let's just say that if the wrong product introduces you to soy, you may decide no health benefit is worth that kind of gustatory abuse! However, most soy products are well designed and extremely appealing. Now that soy is taking its place in the nutrition industry, additional scientific focus will inevitably uncover yet unknown properties of this bean that will probably end up making the six o'clock news.

As of the writing of this book, a new Wake Forest Study designed to single out all of soy's active ingredients is underway.

Armed with a $2.4 million grant from the National Heart, Lung and Blood Institute, the research team, headed by Thomas B. Clarkson, D.V.M., will focus on genistein and daidzein, what they do and how much we need to consume for desired effects. The ratio between these two isoflavones, the optimal use of soy supplements by both men and women and the safety of taking soy will be studied in depth.

Isoflavones and Growth Factor Signaling

Growth factors are molecules that control the reproduction of cells, and they are affected by the presence of estrogen. Scientists have discovered a fascinating link between soy and these factors in tests conducted on people with Osler-Weber-Rendu (OWR) syndrome. OWR is a genetic disorder causing multiple nosebleeds daily. Although the disease is not considered potentially deadly, it can cause loss of blood severe enough to require blood transfusions. At Yale University, OWR patients were placed on a soy protein diet rich in isoflavones. Surprisingly, their nosebleeds dramatically stopped. Scientists realized that the genetic mutations that cause OWR also impair growth factor processes in the human body. Obviously, soy isoflavones were able to fix this malfunction, although how they did so remains unknown. What is of particular interest to researchers is that disorders similar to OWR can also cause potentially fatal diseases like cancer, osteoporosis and heart disease.

Antibiotic and Antifungal Actions of Soy

During a 1997 symposium held in Tucson, Arizona on phytoestrogens research methods, it was reported that soy isoflavones also have significant antibiotic and antifungal properties. According to Terrence Graham, Ph.D., of Ohio State University, the reason soy plants manufacture isoflavones is to protect themselves from environmental perils. Dr. Graham explained that the hormone-like properties of isoflavones not only help to regulate cell reproduction but also function to protect plants from foreign invaders by acting as plant antibiotic and antifungal agents.

Diuretic Effect of Soy Isoflavones

Octavio J. Alda, M.D. has presented evidence that soy isoflavones have an effect similar to the powerful antidiuretic drug called furosemide. Apparently, genistein is a smooth muscle vaso-relaxant, which increases the excretion of sodium, chloride, potassium, magnesium and calcium through the kidneys. Dr. Alda concluded that the soy isoflavonoids offer many benefits in the treatment of heart and kidney disease and may be substituted for prescription loop-diuretics.

Soy's Effect on Kidney Function and Diabetes

Dr. M.G. Gentile, a physician at the Department of Clinical Nutrition and Department of Nephrology at the S. Carol Hospital in Milan, Italy, presented data that lipids (fats) contribute to kidney damage and that correcting lipid abnormalities could slow the progression of chronic kidney disease. Most people are unaware that diets high in animal protein and fat can cause or worsen kidney disease. Soy protein, however, actually works to reduce the protein content of the urine. In one recent study, a vegetarian soy diet caused more than 30 percent of urinary protein excretion and lowered cholesterol by 28 percent. Dr. James W.

Anderson of the VA hospital at the University of Kentucky in Lexington also reported that using forty-two grams of soy protein daily on men with Type II diabetes-related kidney disease resulted in significant kidney improvement. An unexpected bonus of this trial was the discovery that the soy protein diet dramatically reduced (up to 90 percent) the need for insulin in Type II diabetics and that soy protein also increased insulin sensitivity in the same test subjects.

Soy Protein and Gallstone Prevention

We've known for a long time that Western diets play a profound role in the formation of gallstones. In studies, soy protein actually worked to retard the cholesterol crystallization that causes the formation of gallstones. Moreover, test subjects who consumed soy protein experienced a doubling of a particular bile acid that actually dissolves gallstones.

Soy "Smart Bomb" and Leukemia

In February 1999, scientists from the University of Minnesota announced that they had created a "smart bomb," which holds significant potential as a possible cure for the treatment of a common form of childhood leukemia. The smart bomb is comprised of genistein that has been attached to a specific antibody. Genistein was used based on clinical tests, which indicate that it can effectively kill leukemia cells in mice.

Soy: Genital Herpes Buster

Scientists from Johns Hopkins have announced that laboratory tests conducted on mice have shown that an antibody manufactured from soy has the ability to stop the spread of genital herpes. Although currently very expensive, this antibody, scientists point out, could eventually be extracted from soybean plants grown in fields, which would dramatically lower its price.

Genistein and Kaposi's Sarcoma

As we mentioned earlier, genistein has the ability to control the abnormal growth of new blood vessels—required for the survival of a solid tumor. The term that refers to the growth of these blood vessels is angiogenesis, and genistein is considered an antiangiogenesis substance. Angiogenesis also plays a vital role in Kaposi's sarcoma and provides vascular nourishment for any solid tumor that must rely on a new network of blood vessels to grow. Scientists at universities in Heidelberg, Geneva and Helsinki analyzed urine samples from test subjects who were eating a diet rich in soy foods and found that their genistein content was substantially elevated. Genistein has a very powerful antiangiogenesis effect in laboratory tests. The genistein content of the urine of Japanese subjects who eat plenty of soy foods is generally thirty times more concentrated than that of Americans. While the study did not recommend using genistein for Kaposi's sarcoma, which is a common complication of AIDS, it only makes sense that its ability to inhibit angiogenesis may be of benefit.

SOY HEADLINES

Foods for the Future, 1/00: "Research find soy can prevent cancer up to twenty-five percent in laboratory tests."

Science Daily, 10/1/99: "Eating soy can lead to dramatic declines in cholesterol, Wake Forest study shows."

Women's Health, 9/22/99: "FDA approves soy health claims for heart disease."

Science Daily, 1/27/99: "Soy may decrease cancer risks, Wake Forest researchers say. . . ."

Good Housekeeping, 2/97: "There's more and more evidence that soy is something of a natural wonder drug—able to treat menopausal symptoms while helping to lower the risk for heart disease, osteoporosis, and breast cancer."

CNN Headline News, 2/24/97: "Studies show diets rich in soy can lower cholesterol, prevent breast and prostate cancer, and reduce hot flashes in menopausal women."

Health Magazine, 2/3/97: "A particular form of isoflavone in soy could actually defend against many types of cancer."

Boston Globe Magazine, 1/5/97: "Soy products are a good source of protein, iron, potassium, and in some brands, calcium."

Hartford Courant, 1/1/97: "Health professionals suggest incorporating more soy into the daily diet."

Tampa Tribune, 12/16/96: "A diet emphasizing soy foods decreases heart disease and helps prevent hormone-related cancers of the ovaries, prostate and breast."

Soy and Pain Relief

Scientists from Johns Hopkins and two Israeli universities have discovered soybeans may help to control pain. This recent study shows that laboratory rats fed a diet containing soy meal develop significantly less pain after a nerve injury than their counterparts who are on soy-free diets. The study, reported in a recent issue of *Neuroscience Letters,* suggests that diet may have a direct bearing on pain perception. In other words, in this particular case, soy proteins may inhibit the way cells relay pain signals.

Other Health Benefits Linked to Soy

There is evidence that soy can benefit the human body in other ways, most notably by

- preventing impotence by controlling plaque deposits in the penile artery
- possibly extending overall life span
- preventing cholesterol-containing gallstones
- helping to curb alcohol cravings
- acting as a powerful diuretic in cases of heart and kidney disease
- significantly reducing the need for insulin in some diabetics
- enhancing fertility by blocking a male hormone that inhibits semen production

World Soybean Research

The Sixth World Soybean Research Conference (WSRC VI) was held in August 1999, hosting the largest, most notable group of soybean scientists ever assembled under one roof. In addition, the Global Soy Forum '99 (GSF99), which was comprised of representatives from virtually every corner of the world, discussed relevant soy subjects. More than 2,000 leaders in the world soybean industry participated in GSF99. Topics addressed included how the soy industry will respond to the growing nutritional needs of emerging societies and cultures worldwide. In October 1999, the third international symposium on the role of soy in preventing and testing chronic disease, headed by Mark Messina, a world renown soy expert, was also held in Washington, D.C.

Inorganic and Imaginative Soy Products

Soy is so versatile that it has the potential of replacing several chemical compounds currently found in many commercial products. Due to the fact that soy poses no risks to our environment, it provides a marvelous chemical base for several compounds we would never normally associate with soy. For example, soy ink contains no petroleum oil. Soy diesel fuel is nontoxic and biodegradable, which reduces the amount of carbon monoxide and hydrocarbons released in the atmosphere when it is burned. Soy silk may replace the fabric currently made by silkworms and would be both washable and much less costly.

Soy wood adhesives are in the research stage and would create nontoxic glues that would get rid of formaldehyde products that can pollute the environment and pose health risks. Soy plastics could provide us with biodegradable plastics that contain no harmful chemicals and would break down rather than crowd our landfills indefinitely. Soy oil-based candles are in the making, and a new motor oil created with soybean oil is being tested in a cross-country trek across America. This motor oil, used in a Ford F-150 truck, may provide us with improved engine efficiency and corrosion protection while actually reducing emissions and conserving energy—and it's biodegradable.

Note: The United Soybean Board (USB) and the Indiana Soybean Board are wonderful sources of information about soy and can be accessed online at http://www.unitedsoybean.org and http://indianasoybeanboard.com, respectively.

chapter 12

Is Soy Safe?

*"No matter what happens, there's always
somebody who knew it would."*
LONNY STARR

AT THIS POINT, one thing should be perfectly clear. When all is said and done, you will have to be the ultimate judge of what you believe to be safe or not. In our opinion, soy has a remarkable track record and offers all of us, especially women, major health benefits with relatively low risk—something you won't usually find in a pharmaceutical drug. Because soy is the richest source of isoflavones, or natural estrogens, questions concerning its safety inevitably arise. Let's talk about the major concerns surrounding soy use, and then you can make up your own mind.

Can You Eat Too Much Soy?

Like most things, the notion that if a little is good, a whole lot is better does not apply to soy. First of all, avoid eating raw or undercooked soybeans. As mentioned earlier, soybeans contain some undesirable compounds. If you eat over one hundred grams of processed soy foods per day, you could suffer from a glut of estrogens. In other words, an extremely high consumption of soy could result in some unwanted side effects, especially in children or postmenopausal women who are used to lower estrogen levels. Very high doses of soy could also change the menstrual cycle. In fact, clinical data tells us that consuming soy protein at a level of sixty grams per day has been shown to increase menstrual cycle length, while decreasing levels of circulating hormones at the same time. What this suggests is that the way you might react to eating high quantities of soy depends on your particular estrogen status at the time—you can see why there may be cause for concern if too much soy is given to infants or young children. Animal studies have also found that consuming very large amounts of soy in pregnant rats can cause reproductive problems in their offspring. Scientists at Wake Forest University, however, have concluded that plant estrogens do not adversely affect the reproductive systems of males.

A small pilot study mentioned earlier also found that soy increased growth in the breast cells of a test group of women taking a soy protein supplement. Ironically, consuming too little soy may also stimulate breast cell growth, although there are no human studies to date confirming this. Some experts recommend using doses at the higher end of the scale for therapeutic reasons (much the same way a drug is used) and smaller ones for prevention. All in all, what we do know leads us to believe that in most cases moderation is the key. Optimal soy consumption should normally fall between thirty-five and sixty grams of soy food per day. Getting this amount by eating traditional soy foods like tofu may be difficult. Soy protein powders that you can add to foods or use in shakes make targeted soy consumption much easier.

A Word About Current Anti-Soy Sentiments

Recently, some studies have surfaced that suggest that eating too much tofu or other soy products with isoflavones may cause brain cells to die off. These studies are based on the fact that soy isoflavones (genistein in particular) inhibit DNA replication. If you remember, this is one of the ways in which genistein helps to fight cancerous tumors. Simply stated, these studies claim that this same mechanism can also kill off healthy cells in the brain and other parts of the body. The studies have sparked a rash of soy warnings that have people wondering what to believe.

Let us just begin by saying that you can find negative studies on virtually every beneficial compound including beta carotene, vitamin C, vitamin E, calcium, etc. Studies exist that challenge the validity of practically any nutrient, and a few of these studies even conclude that certain nutrients pose a health risk. Frequently, however, the results of these isolated trials are based on using extreme dosages, and our core belief that moderation in all things is the key to good health applies here.

As far as the new "anti-soy" studies are concerned, one has to question their methodology and their interpretation. What we do know is that the overwhelming consensus among nutritionists is that soy foods are good for us. Moreover, hundreds of studies confirm that the soybean is full of positive therapeutic properties. To turn away from the extraordinary health benefits of soy due to a few scant studies that are critical of soy and then to throw a steak on the barbeque is rather ludicrous. It's also important to keep in mind that soy foods are nothing new. Asian cultures have consumed several servings of tofu and other soy foods daily for millenia. As far as we know, there is no scientific data suggesting that these people have been mentally compromised in any way.

Clearly, soy compounds are powerful and multifaceted biochemicals that should be treated with respect and used judiciously. It is precisely for this reason that we encourage eating whole phytoestrogenic foods over taking soy constituents in isolated supplement forms. This is not because we think that isolated soy supplements are dangerous or ineffective, but rather we have no way of knowing exactly how they affect the human body. Soy compounds such as phytates, trypsin inhibitors and isoflavones may have adverse effects on healthy tissue if misused, and more research needs to be done. Whole soy foods, however, have centuries of benefits to back them up, and we have no doubt that the soybean was designed for human consumption.

Like any plant food, however, using soy in extreme doses by assuming that if a little is good, more must be better is not wise. Moreover, be aware that as the popularity of soy foods escalates, more rival studies will emerge. This is where good old common sense comes into play. The facts speak for themselves. We should also add that for a society that routinely overdoses on aspartame, white sugar, olestra, hydrogenated fats and cholesterol, learning to eat soy foods regularly is one of the single most health-promoting dietary changes we can make.

Soy Formulas for Infants

Soy-based infant formulas were first marketed in the 1960s and provided mothers of allergic infants a welcome alternative to cow's milk. The use of these formulas has been on the rise until recently. Soy-based infant formulas are quite similar to other infant formulas except that a soy protein isolate powder instead of cow's milk is used as a base. Fats and carbohydrates are also added to simulate the fluid texture of milk.

Currently, the use of soy for infants has sparked some ongoing scientific debate. However, there have been very few reports of negative side effects associated with thousands of infants who have taken soy formulas over the last few decades. The possibility that these formulas might harm the sexual development of children is the major concern and has been linked with the early onset of puberty in developed countries. Naturally, when it comes to premature puberty, there could be many possible contributing factors. Nevertheless, the controversy has initiated a new inquiry into the safety of phytoestrogens for infants.

Dr. Kenneth Setchell addresses this concern, and he points out that the potential for creating a hormonal imbalance with soy formulas exists. Based on average figures, an infant would normally consume fifteen to thirty-five milligrams of isoflavones daily through formula supplementation. The excretion of these isoflavones has been confirmed in urine samples of tested babies. Those levels, however, are considerably lower than would be seen in an adult consuming even less isoflavones. This suggests that the infant digestive tract does not assimilate isoflavones the same way as an adult. Dr. Setchell is also quick to reiterate that we lack the data to make an accurate assessment at this time. While the general consensus is that infants should only use soy-based formulas in cases of cow's milk allergies, there is no substantial reason to prohibit their use. Because of bad publicity, a 35 percent reduction in sales of soy infant formulas has occurred over the last two years.

Nursing Mothers and Soy Consumption

Studies tell us that normally the phytoestrogen concentration in human breast milk is negligible unless the lactating mother has consumed soy foods. A tenfold increase of this concentration in breast milk has been seen when the mother consumes soy foods, although the total amount of these isoflavone compounds is still relatively low when compared to soy infant formulas. According to available data, scientists feel that there is little reason to be concerned about the isoflavone exchange in breast milk from mother to infant. These compounds are seen as extremely weak and are not thought to cause any significant side effects in the nursing baby. Therefore, nursing mothers can still eat soy foods in reasonable amounts. Soy foods are an excellent source of protein and can supply a rich array of needed nutrients during lactation, when dietary needs are dramatically increased.

Isoflavone Supplements: A Good Idea?

As nutritional supplement companies jump on the soy band-wagon, the safety of taking isoflavones in pill form has become a hot topic. Ideally, the best way to benefit from soy phytoestrogens is to include isoflavone-rich soy foods in our daily diets. Regarding taking isoflavones in pill form, caution is the general rule among most scientists due to the fact that we just don't know whether they are actually effective or safe. Genistein, for example, has the potential to be toxic if taken in high doses, while daidzein operates differently and seems to be nontoxic.

The issue of what happens to soy isoflavones that come from food sources as they pass through the intestinal tract is also pertinent. When you take an isolated isoflavone supplement, you bypass the process by which isoflavones are naturally absorbed and assimilated. Moreover, the synergy between isoflavones and other phytosterols found in soy will most likely prove to be of much more therapeutic value than using one single isolated soy compound such as genistein or daidzein. By assuming that only one of the primary chemical constituents of soy is therapeutically valuable, so-called "inactive" compounds that can play a vital role in the human body are eliminated. Isolated, mimicked or potentiated drug compounds are not equivalent to the whole plant or herb. Refining or synthesizing various compounds can create toxicity. In other words, because they are presented to the body in an unnatural state, stripped of other substances that act as balancing agents, these isolated compounds are not readily accepted by body systems.

Simply said, Nature usually knows best. It is important to remember that unlike the potent, quick and sometimes dangerous effects of synthetic drugs or analogs, foods like soy and other plant agents work more slowly. The bottom line is that while most drugs act rapidly, with stronger action, shorter lasting effects, and more potentially dangerous side effects, foods like soy take more time, have a gentler action with effects that can be long-lasting, and pose much less risk. While most physicians rely on synthetic drugs, more and more of them are recognizing the value of therapies designed by Mother Nature.

The potential side effects of single compound supplements are another concern. Because we are treading on new ground, no one can definitely state whether isoflavone supplements are safe or not. The dilemma here is that no one knows how much is too much when using an isolated compound extracted from soy in a supplement form. The ratio of genistein to daidzein in the soybean is also an issue. Each component of the bean as it relates to other components is missing from supplement products. As data emerges, we may discover that isoflavone supplements can serve a very valuable purpose, especially if you are allergic to soy foods or have trouble developing a taste for them. At this point, however, taking isoflavone supplements may still be premature. Hopefully, in the near future, their use will be scientifically supported. At this point, we just don't know.

YOUNG WOMEN AND SOY

Should an adolescent girl be concerned about eating soy? One study published in the *British Journal of Nutrition* examined the hormonal effects of isoflavones on fifteen healthy premenopausal women for over nine months. Researchers found that the women's progesterone levels were affected and their menstrual cycles were lengthened. Concerns center on possible negative changes in breast cells or reproductive functions of young women. Keep in mind, however, that Japanese girls have eaten soy for generations without any apparent negative side effects.

Our feeling is that common sense needs to prevail here. Exchanging a greasy cheeseburger with fries or a hydrogenated fat- and sugar-loaded doughnut for a tofu shake would certainly be a health improvement. Again, moderation needs to prevail until we know more. Soy foods can also help a young girl with safe and nutritious weight management.

Infertility Issues and Soy

While some studies have suggested that eating soy in very excessive quantities may cause infertility, other tests found that soy isoflavones may actually enhance male fertility. The anti-estrogen activity of soy isoflavones may positively impact blood levels of luteinizing hormone (LH), which is required for sperm to produce normally. Men in Japan typically receive between forty and sixty milligrams of genistein daily, while American men consume less than one milligram per day. Eating appropriate amounts of soy may help to boost the synthesis of steroid hormones like testosterone, which could better chances for reproduction. The watchword here is not to eat soy in excess. The Asian model tells us that soy consumption kept within reasonable ranges should not cause fertility problems and may even increase the chances of conception.

Allergies to Soy

A significant number of people are allergic to soy protein, which is ranked eleventh among foods that can cause allergic reactions. Keep in mind, however, that people who are allergic to cow's milk, which is a more prevalent food allergy, often use soy milk. Soy allergies are usually seen in younger people and are considered uncommon among adults. If you eat soy and develop skin rashes, gas, facial swelling, difficulty swallowing or even fainting, you may be allergic to soy. Infants who develop either a soy or cow's milk allergy may have diarrhea, vomiting, irritability, chronic rashes, asthma or runny nose. If you are allergic to soy, you need to avoid the following:

- hydrolyzed vegetable protein
- isolated soy protein
- textured soy protein (TSP)
- miso

- natto
- soy cheese
- soy protein concentrates
- soy nuts
- soy oil
- yuba
- tofu products

- okara
- soy sauces (teriyaki, tamari, etc.)
- soy isolates and flours
- soy grits
- tempeh
- soy beverages

Note: Avoid lecithin if it is made from soy oil. Remember that soy meal may be a hidden ingredient of a number of industrial products, including inks, soap, cosmetics, etc. If you are in doubt, call the manufacturer.

The particular way in which soy foods are processed can also determine their allergy potential. Fermented soy products such as miso, tempeh, shoyu, tofu and natto are generally considered less allergenic than raw soybeans. Soy sauce rarely causes problems in that it is usually consumed in such small amounts and is low in soy protein. It is the protein component or the fermentation process of soy that is responsible for its allergenic properties. If you have a soy allergy, use flaxseed oil as a source of phytoestrogens. Other possible sources of phytoestrogens are listed in chapter one. You may also want to look into using natural progesterone cream for natural hormone balancing.

A web site dedicated to soy allergy sufferers that contains a list of foods and other products that are soy-free can be found at http://www.geocities.com/HotSprings/4620.

New Hope for Those Allergic to Soy

In 1991, Professor Tadashi Ogawa of the University of Tokushima School of Medicine isolated the soybean allergenic protein, Glym Bd 30K. Ogawa and his team found that Glym Bd 30K was the most strongly and frequently serum-recognized protein among people with allergic rashes. Professor Ogawa has developed a simple technique to produce hypoallergenic soybean products for soybean sensitive people, and he has developed a centrifugation-based technique that removes more than 90 percent of the offending protein from soybean extract adjusted for ion and pH levels. For more information, contact:

Professor Tadashi Ogawa
Department of Nutrition
University of Tokushima School of Medicine
Tel: 81-886-31-3111
Fax: 81-886-33-0771

chapter 13

Guidelines for Great Hormonal Health

"The body is a test tube. You have to put in exactly the right ingredients to get the best reaction out of it."
JACK YOUNGBLOOD

TOM ROBBINS ONCE said, "To be or not to be isn't the question. The question is how to prolong being." While that may be true, adding years to our lives makes no sense if poor health and debility compromise our existence. What we choose to put in our mouths determines, to a great extent, the quality of our years. Keep in mind that until the turn of the twentieth century, Western medicine focused on the use of various plants and foods for the treatment of disease.

There is no question that we live in a time when the demand for products that are plant-based has dramatically escalated. A pervasive disillusionment with conventional medicine and its "medicate everything" approach is spreading throughout the public. The need to know and to have the right to use dietary therapies has dramatically increased over the last twenty years. While no one wants to dispute the lifesaving value of antibiotics, steroidal anti-inflammatories etc., drugs are routinely over-prescribed and pose significant health risks as well. By contrast, phytonutrients are naturally accepted by the body and infinitely safer. Many of them also have the ability to heal and correct, an action which usually lies beyond the capability of synthetic drugs, which mask or simply treat the symptoms rather than the cause of disease. The soybean and other plants and herbs offer us some viable dietary solutions.

A Millennial Medical Revolution

Ironically, in the midst of modern medicine capable of transplanting organs, the American public is turning away from pharmaceutical solutions in droves. We are in the dawn of a revolution in health care that most physicians are barely aware of. The twenty-first century will inevitably see the most dramatic reinvention of medical practices in over 150 years. We would like to be able to say that all doctors are seeing the light. The truth is, however, that most of them won't until they feel the heat—the heat created by a public who want to be apprized of all of their health options and who are coming over to natural medicine by the droves. We were surprised to learn that the annual number of visits to alternative care practitioners now exceeds those to primary care physicians.

The consequences of pollution, poor nutrition and our unfortunate reliance on prescription and over-the-counter drugs have forced us as a society to re-examine the value of natural, safe therapies. Moreover, more and more scientific evidence continues to mount supporting the validity of herbs and the profound effect of diet, vitamins and minerals on disease prevention and treatment. A whole host of very viable, tried and true alternative treatment options exist. Consider this: After founding the Bio-Brain Center in Princeton, New Jersey, Dr. Karl Pfeiffer stated, "For every drug that benefits a patient, there is a natural substance that can achieve the same effect."

We live in a society that is quick to medicate itself without looking into the whys and wherefores of disease. Dr. Malcom Todd, past president of the American Medical Association, put it best when he said, "Thus far physicians have shown little objective interest in promoting health and preventive care. We actually have a disease-oriented cure system, rather than a health-oriented care system in this country today."

Diet: The Forgotten Solution

Today, we know that up to 70 percent of certain cancers can be attributed to our diets. Moreover, eating an excess of animal foods coupled with high sugar consumption has simultaneously increased our risk of several degenerative diseases. We believe that if we ate enough raw fruits, vegetables, legumes and whole grains, we could significantly mitigate the effects of the animal fats and protein we eat. It's all about balance, and some of our greatest weapons against cancer are powerful phytonutrients found in fruits and vegetables. Unfortunately, the medical community and other agencies have not fostered and funded campaigns strong enough to get this message across to the American public. Present assumptions are that efforts to bring about dietary changes in the public are doomed for failure, so many people turn to chemical alternatives.

Plant Phytochemicals: The Missing Link in the American Diet

Just a few years ago, no one even knew that phytochemicals existed. Today, with the routine emergence of new plant compounds, scientists are turning their attention to the marvelous medicinal compounds that Mother Nature has hidden in simple foods. The general consensus is that phytochemicals hold profound therapeutic promises that go beyond the action of simple vitamins and minerals. At this writing, scientists are in the process of isolating these remarkable natural chemicals in an attempt to use them therapeutically for the treatment of disease.

Mountains of research data confirm that a diet high in vegetables and fruits is cancer-protective. This is because fruits and vegetables contain an impressive array of powerful substances that work to inhibit carcinogenic pathways. Some of these phytochemicals include carotenoids such as carotene, vitamin C, vitamin E, selenium, and dietary fiber, in addition to other beneficial nutrients that come in the form of dithiolthiones, isothiocyanates, indoles, phenols and phytoestrogens. Phytonutrients have the distinct ability to protect us on a cellular level from virtually any cancer-causing agent.

The Value of Isoflavones: Why Isn't the Word Spreading?

We've established the fact that the soybean is capable of inhibiting the action of estradiol in women. In light of the fact that isoflavones have so many significant therapeutic benefits for women, it's disturbing that the medical community has failed to get the word out. The profound disease-preventing capabilities of soy isoflavones rank with some of our most powerful medicines, yet physicians rarely acknowledge their properties. Moreover, a vast variety of phytonutrients found in fruits, vegetables and herbs are only now beginning to emerge as scientifically credible phyto-pharmaceuticals. After reviewing the multitude of studies conducted on soy compounds, it is safe to say that American consumers (especially women) should be aggressively incorporating soy foods into their diets.

Moreover, cruciferous plants, which include broccoli and cabbage, contain substances called indoles that can also keep bad estrogen in check. Of equal importance is that dietary fiber may also interfere with the development of breast tumors by mitigating the effect of estrogen when plant lignans are chemically changed in the colon by friendly bacteria. Simply stated, foods that contain high concentrations of indoles and other compounds can help protect tissue from hormonal carcinogens by inactivating them. Isn't it amazing how all of our body systems interrelate to help protect us from disease? Unfortunately, every part of the body needs to be in tiptop shape for optimal protection. For example, if your colon is compromised, your system of defense can break down.

The following guidelines offered in this chapter are essentially the same for breast cancer prevention as they are for menopause or PMS relief. The bottom line is that one set of parameters is emerging that promotes good health and protects us from disease. We should eat a lot more fresh fruits, vegetables, whole grains and legumes, and we should use high quality sources of protein and good fats, as well as avoid white flour, white sugar, processed foods, caffeine and alcohol.

Increase Your Soy Consumption

Both young and old Japanese women eat from 2.5 to 3.5 ounces of tofu every day. We believe that the Japanese model is our best bet for optimal soy use. One could argue that you may need a certain amount of soy for antioxidant protection, a different amount for breast cancer prevention and still another for menopause. The following guidelines, however, are based on the credo of moderation in all things and on the belief that in most cases, eating too much or too little soy is not necessarily a good thing. If you're not used to eating soy, start with 10 grams a day and build up from there to avoid any possible intestinal gas or stomach upset. You may find that you cannot tolerate soy or that you are allergic to it, in which case, you will need to use the other nutrient strategies covered in this chapter.

Generally speaking, try to eat no less than twenty-five grams and no more than sixty grams of soy protein daily. Remember that a minimum of twenty-five grams of soy protein daily is required for effective cholesterol benefits. While the phytoestrogen content of soy foods varies considerably for each product, one or two servings of tofu, soybeans or soy milk a day is equivalent to the normal soy intake of Asian women—this includes approximately thirty-five milligrams of isoflavones.

Claire Hasler, University of Illinois nutritionist and expert on soy, recommends finding your ideal soy intake based on your protein needs. For example, she explains, "A 150-pound (68 kilograms) male would need 0.8 kilograms protein per gram of ideal body weight. Assuming that [this man is at his] ideal body weight, then [he] would require, for general health maintenance, about 55 grams of protein per day." In terms of measuring soy protein, the FDA is proposing an assay method that detects soy in both raw and heat-processed products. The FDA is currently reviewing public comment on the value of this method.

What to Look for on Soy Food Labels

First, look for protein content—it's the protein component of soy that contains the necessary isoflavones. If the product you are checking is low in protein (such as soy sauce), it will be lacking or entirely missing isoflavones. The words *soy protein concentrate* may or may not indicate a good isoflavone source, depending on how the product was processed. Look for labels that actually list terms like isolated soy protein, soy protein isolate or textured soy protein. Also, as mentioned earlier, many products can now post an FDA approved comment on their soy protein content if they meet the FDA's minimum requirements. These labels will explain the relationship between soy protein and a reduced risk for heart disease, and they will give the amount of soy protein per serving in the product.

Remember also that sometimes meat substitute products made of textured soy protein may be missing isoflavones due to processing techniques. Mark Messina, Ph.D. and coauthor of *The Simple Soybean and Your Health,* warns that the kind of soy protein often found in soy burgers and related products is not a good source of phytoestrogens. The use of alcohols to modify the color, flavor and smell of soy may also remove its isoflavone content. Dr. Messina points out that these products offer a wonderful, high-quality protein alternative to meat but do little to manipulate hormones.

In addition, just because a food has the word *soy* in its title doesn't mean the food affords us significant health benefits. For example, you won't find any of the cancer-protective properties we've talked about in soy sauce or soybean oil. In fact, soybean oil that has been hydrogenated is not recommended at all. Remember it's the soy protein in soy that contains isoflavones. If in doubt about a product, call the manufacturer, or you may be wasting your money.

Best Soy Sources of Isoflavones

Ideally, if we are looking to soy foods as our only source of isoflavones, we need to make sure we consume at least thirty-five milligrams of isoflavones per day (refer to the isoflavone content charts in a later section for more information). Most soy foods contain one to two milligrams of genistein per gram. Below are examples of some soy foods and their isoflavone count:

- One ounce of soy chips or nuts contains forty-two milligrams of isoflavones.
- One hundred grams of soy flour contain fifty isoflavones.
- Four ounces of tofu contain eighty milligrams of isoflavones.
- Eight ounces of raw soy milk contain fifty milligrams of isoflavones.

Foods to incorporate into the diet include tofu, soy milk, soy chips, miso, soy flour, soy protein drinks, soy nuts and spreads. You can put soy powder into any baking recipe. Tofu can be whipped into dips, sauces, mashed potatoes, spreads, desserts, fillings, etc. (refer to recipe section). And now, even popular breakfast cereals from makers like Kellogg's are available with soy as a primary ingredient. (Other foods will inevitably follow suit.)

Soy protein concentrate can be an excellent source of isoflavones. Genistein is the primary isoflavone found in soy protein concentrate. The amount of genistein present in soy protein concentrate averages from 0.48 to 1.51 milligrams per gram. Be aware that all soy protein products do not contain isoflavones. Some isoflavones are actually removed through processing, so look for isoflavone content on the label, and if none is listed, call the manufacturer.

New Soy Database

A new database on soy products for consumers will give all of us access to important health reports concerning soy. Nutritionists at the U.S. Department of Agriculture (USDA) have finally recognized that isoflavones have antioxidant effects that can potentially reduce heart disease and cancer risks. These nutritionists are now working with Iowa State University to create a list of 128 soy-containing and related foods. It will be the first database available on isoflavones, with information gleaned from hundreds of scientific articles. Additional information, which is the result of extensive sampling and analysis of soy foods, will also be listed. You can access this information on the USDA web site at http://www.nal.usda.gov/fnic/foodcomp/Data/isoflav/isoflav.html.

This new database results from a joint project involving the USDA's food composition laboratory and nutrient data laboratory and Iowa State University's Department of Food Science and Nutrition. The project was initiated after a 1998 FDA proposal to permit food manufacturers to make health claims for soy-related products. Consequently, soy foods will now be outfitted with new labels listing their health benefits. The FDA ruling is based on data supporting the fact that soy protein may reduce the risk of heart disease. Soy foods may also be cited as cancer inhibitors.

The new soy database will contain files giving isoflavone values, references and studies. Refer to the reference section of this book for this new isoflavone-content chart.

Nutrients that Complement Soy Isoflavones

The ideal protocol for maintaining hormonal health incorporates not only soy but also various other nutrients with impressive track records. Read on to learn which natural supplements support and complement soy protein for optimal health and vitality.

Curcumin and Quercitin

New data support the addition of curcumin and quercitin as isoflavone potentiators. Studies have found that adding curcumin (found in turmeric root) to genistein greatly boosted its anti-estrogenic effects. Curcumin and genistein worked together with synergistic actions that inhibited the growth of human breast cancer cells that were created by exposure to powerful estrogenic pesticides. Scientists concluded that the combination of curcumin and genistein in the diet have the potential to prevent hormone-related cancers that are stimulated by our environment. Quercitin, a bioflavonoid and powerful antioxidant, has a similar effect. Researchers recommend taking 500 milligrams of quercitin and 600 milligrams of curcumin daily.

Natural Progesterone

In his book, *What Your Doctor May Not Tell You about Menopause,* John R. Lee, a physician, discusses hormone balance and natural progesterone. Natural progesterone (made from wild yams or soybeans) has active ingredients that on a molecular level closely resemble the progesterone produced in the female body. By using high quality natural progesterone creams, the ill effects of estrogen we discussed in chapter one can be safely modulated.

Remember that when estrogen is properly opposed by progesterone, several beneficial effects are obtained (refer to chapter one). Dr. Lee began recommending progesterone for women with menopausal symptoms in 1979. After ten years of prescribing natural progesterone, he realized that many of his patients who were using it did not experience fibrocystic breasts, fibroid tumors, thyroid deficiencies, osteoporosis or difficulty maintaining pregnancies to term. In addition, in her book *Dr. Susan Love's Hormone Book,* Dr. Susan Love talks about the value of creating hormonal balance with natural progesterone.

It is possible that progesterone may even be more important than estrogen in maintaining bone density after menopause. Remember that progesterone production stops altogether after menopause. Interestingly, progesterone levels dramatically increase during pregnancy. This may explain why some women who may have been estrogen dominant feel unusually good for nine months. During gestation, progesterone is produced in large quantities by the placenta (up to ten times the normal amount) to hold the pregnancy. Using an effective natural progesterone cream can greatly contribute to opposing estrogen in a safe way when you're not pregnant. Many of the actions of natural progesterone listed below are just the opposite of estrogen-driven symptoms.

Therapeutic Applications of Natural Progesterone

Natural progesterone is certainly valuable for many reasons. The following are a summarized list of progesterone's health benefits. Natural progesterone

- is necessary for the survival and development of the fetus
- helps to prevent osteoporosis
- is needed for the proper production of adrenal hormones
- works to stabilize blood sugar
- has a natural diuretic action
- prevents salt retention
- acts as an antidepressant
- helps prevent the formation of fibrocystic breasts

- enhances thermogenesis (the burning of fat)
- contributes to regulating the thyroid gland
- enhances libido
- helps protect the uterus and breasts from malignancies
- contributes to blood clotting mechanisms
- is a precursor of corticosterones
- helps to protect against breast cancer
- normalizes zinc and copper levels
- maintains the secretory endometrium

Combining natural progesterone with the action of soy isoflavones may be the perfect duo for HRT substitution. A report in *Gynecological Endocrinology* stated that using natural progesterone is appealing due to the fact that it poses no risks to liver health, which is a major worry with prescription hormones.

Natural Progesterone and Safety Concerns

Natural progesterone is one of the safest supplements available. In contrast to synthetic progestins, this form of progesterone has little or no side effects. Some women may experience an initial reaction to introducing natural progesterone, a phenomenon that involves an estrogen response. In these cases, estrogen-related symptoms may temporarily become worse. If this occurs, natural progesterone should be continued or dosages adjusted until hormonal balance is achieved. Incidental spotting between periods may occur but is usually resolved within three to five cycles. The use of natural progesterone has not been linked to any form of human cancer. Combining natural progesterone with other drugs has not resulted in any known interference or alteration. No adverse effects of natural progesterone have been reported on the developing fetus of pregnant women, unlike the synthetic progesterone counterparts. Its safe use, however, in pregnant or nursing mothers has not been clinically documented.

After Dr. Lee's findings about natural progesterone began to circulate, all kinds of different creams hit the market. The cream can be used by pre- and postmenopausal women to avoid estrogen-stimulated disorders, including osteoporosis, or to provide some estrogenic effects after menopause. Dr. Lee reminds women that it is very important to read product labels when purchasing natural progesterone cream. Just because a label may list wild yam extract as an ingredient doesn't mean it contains real natural progesterone.

Natural progesterone is delivered through the skin (up to 85 percent of oral applications are excreted by the liver). Rub one quarter to one half teaspoon on vascular areas where veins are visible (neck, top of hands, ankles, etc.) one to two times daily for the last two weeks of the menstrual cycle (rotate sites weekly). Look for natural progesterone creams with 0.4 to 1 percent natural progesterone content.

Cruciferous Vegetables

Cruciferous is the technical term for a group of plants whose four petal flowers resemble a cross. These vegetables are a part of the cabbage family and include arugula, bok choy, broccoli, broccoli sprouts, Brussels sprouts, cabbage, cauliflower, Swiss chard, collards, kale, kohlrabi, mustard greens, radishes, rutabaga, turnips, turnip greens and watercress. Twenty years ago, studies found that people who ate significant amounts of these vegetables had a decreased risk for cancer. Early in the 1990s, researchers discovered two sulfur-containing compounds in cruciferous vegetables (dithiolthiones and isothiocyanates) that are able to increase the activity of enzymes involved in detoxifying some carcinogens. A compound called Indole-3-carbinol was also found to affect estrogen metabolism and is thought to exert a protective effect against estrogen-related cancers. Cruciferous vegetables are nutrient powerhouses and contain fiber and vitamin C and beta-carotene.

As far as the estrogen effect goes, every woman should be eating cruciferous vegetables on a regular basis. The Asian diet is not only high in soy but in cabbage consumption as well, suggesting that the combination of a cruciferous vegetable with soy makes for a powerful and healthy duo. Indole-3-carbinol has already accrued some impressive data backing its use as an effective estrogen blocker. In a study at the Institute for Hormone Research in New York, twelve healthy volunteers (seven men and five women) were given daily doses of 350–500 milligrams of indole-3-carbinol, which is equivalent to ten to twelve ounces of raw cabbage or Brussels sprouts. After a week, indole-3-carbinol had converted estrogen into a metabolite other than the one linked to the formation of cancer. This effect was later duplicated using a cruciferous vegetable extract in a larger group of women.

Broccoli also contains something called sulforaphane, which scientists at the Johns Hopkins School of Medicine in Baltimore found increases the production of enzymes such as quinone reductase and glutathione transferase—both of which work to detoxify the effects of cancer-causing chemicals in the human body.

Consume one or more daily servings of raw or steamed cruciferous vegetables as part of a diet centered on fresh vegetables and fruits, whole grains, legumes, raw nuts, seeds, soy and related products. As time goes on, we are discovering other impressive anticancerous compounds in fresh fruits and vegetables, such as lycopene in tomatoes. What this tells us is that we need to dramatically increase our intake of fresh vegetables and fruits (such as tomatoes, dark lettuce, green peppers, carrots, fresh citrus fruits, apples, melons, etc.). Evidence is mounting that individuals who eat five servings daily of fruits and vegetables, including some cruciferous vegetables, cut their risk for cancer by half when compared to those who consume one serving or less.

Garlic and onions also contain sulfur compounds that inhibit the biological processes that allow cancer cells to replicate.

A Word on Indole-3-Carbinol Supplements

As we previously discussed, the active ingredient of indole-3-carbinol helps to transform dangerous estrogen into more benign

LOSE THE BAD FATS AND USE THE GOOD ONES

Many health experts (including the authors of this book) believe that it is not so much what we're eating that makes us sick, but what we're not eating. Such is the case with fats. The American diet is top-heavy in certain types of fat and contains practically none of others. This gross imbalance is now thought to be linked to rising cancer and heart disease rates and may explain why cultures that eat diets high in animal fats do not always have high rates of heart disease or breast cancer. In other words, it's not just a case of eliminating certain fats. There's a piece of the puzzle that's missing. Keep in mind also that fat cells abound in breast tissue and have an impact on estrogen metabolism. The kind of fat that is stored in your breast depends on the kind you eat. It can either work to mitigate the effects of estrogen or aggravate them.

forms and has been recognized by the National Cancer Institute. It also has been shown to stop the growth of breast cancer cells by inhibiting the action of a specific enzyme.

Any woman who is at high risk for breast cancer, or women who cannot become accustomed to eating cruciferous vegetables, should take an indole-3-carbinol supplement on a daily basis. Many health professionals recommend taking 300–600 milligrams daily.

The Dangers of Transfatty Acids

Margarines often contain compounds called transfatty acids that are created when liquid oil is converted to a solid stick. These artificially formed acids have been linked with increased artery disease as well as breast cancer. Terms like *hydrogenated* or *partially hydrogenated* found on food labels usually signal the presence of transfatty acids and are commonly included in a wide variety of cookies, crackers, muffins, pies, etc. Granted, all of us will inevitably consume some transfatty oils. However, it's wise to keep them on the low end of your fat ratio or try to avoid them altogether.

Omega-6 Fatty Acids: Culprit Fats

While this is still a debatable subject, we believe that limiting omega-6 fats is a good idea for anyone concerned with estrogen-stimulated symptoms. Omega-6 fats are polyunsaturated fats, and while they have been touted in the past as heart healthy, their increased consumption over the past several years has been associated with rising breast cancer rates. A study published in a leading medical journal found that using polyunsaturated fat increased the risk of breast cancer by almost 70 percent. Many people switched from butter to margarine and corn oil because they thought these foods were healthier. Omega-6 fats include oils like corn, cottonseed, peanut and grapeseed oil—even soybean oil falls into this category. To make matters more complicated, polyunsaturated fats are in just about every prepared or packaged food you pick up at the grocery.

Omega-3 and Omega-9 Fats: Hormone Friendly

By contrast, omega-3 fatty acids work to block the estrogen effect and have wonderful cardiovascular benefits as well. Looking at the diet of certain Eskimo women who ate plenty of fish rich with omega-3 fatty acids and had a zero incidence of breast cancer led to the discovery of this link. Studies show that these remarkable fatty acids not only work to prevent the formation of cancerous tumors but can even shrink human breast cancer tumors and inhibit their spread throughout the body. This is impressive data indeed and tells us again that fat can be a powerful nutrient if it's the right kind. Americans don't eat a lot of coldwater fish, and they use fats that are typically high in omega-6 fatty acids. Can you see why our fat consumption imbalances have wreaked havoc with our health? We eat plenty of the bad fats but hardly any of the good ones. You may want to consider adding a fish oil supplement to your diet. Naturally, consuming certain seafood on a regular basis is a great way to get the omega-3 fatty acids, but realistically, many women will fail to eat enough fish and need to consider appropriate supplementation of omega-3 fatty acids at 100 to 1,500 milligrams daily.

Use omega-9 fats for cooking and in salad dressings. Omega-9 fats are monounsaturated fats like olive oil. Several studies on the books suggest that olive oil can actually protect breast tissue against the formation of cancerous tumors. When it comes to saturated fats found in animal foods, remember that the human body makes its primary hormones from dietary cholesterol. Therefore, while we need to watch our cholesterol intake, we shouldn't eliminate it altogether. Moderation is the key. There are many health professionals who believe that eating animal fats with sweet or starchy foods at the same time can be detrimental. When insulin levels rise after a meal comprised of animal protein, fats and carbohydrates (like steak with white potatoes, rice, breads, and dessert), you have a biochemical reaction that can increase the risk of obesity, artery disease and even breast cancer. If you want to eat animal protein with its accompanying fat, it may be wise to limit the consumption of any carbohydrate foods in the same meal. In this manner, blood sugar levels will not rise at the same time blood fat levels do.

Flaxseed Oil

Flaxseed oil may lower the production of potentially dangerous estrogens by blocking some of their tumor initiating effects. In fact, according to a 1993 article published in *Clinical Endocrinology Metabolism,* flaxseed oil enhances progesterone/estradiol ratios during menstruation. It can be taken as a supplement or used as a liquid oil in dishes such as salads. You should take approximately thirty grams of flaxseed oil per day, especially if you are allergic to soy foods.

A Word on the Fat Content of Soy

As far as the fat content of soy goes, some soy foods (like tofu) contain a fair amount of fat. This fat, however, is unsaturated and considered healthy. Remember that soy foods combine an excellent source of protein with beneficial fat, creating a perfect dietary combination. Our overreaction to fat content of any kind in foods has led to a gross misconception. Fats as part of highly nutritious and desirable foods like soy can play an integral role in health maintenance. Fat is necessary for the production of hormones and also helps us to stay trim (yes, you heard us right). Good fats balanced with good protein and carbohydrates from whole grains and plants result in a well-functioning human machine. It is the addition of white sugar, white flour, and other highly refined foods that makes fat a problem. In addition, we need to use fats that have a good track record—like olive oil and even butter when used in moderation. Butter is beginning to regain its reputation as a cholesterol-friendly food if used properly. As we mentioned earlier, it is the artificially hardened margarines touted as being so heart-friendly that truly make us sick.

Become Fiber-Friendly

Scientists have discovered that estrogen levels go down when sufficient amounts of wheat bran are added to the diet of women. Because wheat bran is primarily an insoluble fiber, this makes good sense. Insoluble fibers can bind much more readily to substances like estrogen in the bowel, thereby eliminating them from the body more efficiently. Most women rarely associate constipation with estrogen levels. The link, however, is a valid one. Moreover, if you are taking prescription estrogens, keep in mind that dietary fiber affects the way these hormones will be metabolized in your liver.

Clearly, women seem much more susceptible to constipation than men and are frequently dependent on laxatives. In the United States alone, the annual sales of laxatives and stool softeners amounts to over $500 million annually. Simply stated, if your bowel is not eliminating waste efficiently, you will never enjoy optimal health, no matter what supplements you are taking. Adding fiber to your diet is one of the simplest ways to remedy constipation.

Fiber helps decrease transit time (the time required for food to make the journey from the mouth to excretion). As we mentioned earlier, fiber also makes the stool heavier, thereby expediting the removal of cancer-causing substances, including estrogen, from the body. Remember that because waste matter can sit in the bowel for twenty-four hours or more, estrogen can be reabsorbed into the body. Fiber can help to prevent this phenomenon. Breast cells need estrogen to grow. If you decrease the amount of circulating estrogen, you decrease your risk of breast cancer. Studies have found a relationship between the fiber content of stool and lower estrogen levels in the body.

Remember that soybeans are legumes, which can help promote regularity. There are approximately 6 grams of fiber per cup of cooked soybeans. There is 1 gram of fiber in 4 ounces of tofu, and there are 4.3 grams of fiber in 3.5 ounces of defatted soy flour. Soy flour is created from the hull and seed of the soybean. Soy flour helps to decrease transit time and promote better elimination, lowers bad cholesterol and even helps to stabilize blood sugar levels in people with diabetes. Eating plenty of vegetable fiber, grain fiber and fiber from fruits and berries has been associated with low levels of several hormones including testosterone, estrone, androstenedione and free estradiol. One good rule of thumb is to eat enough fiber that your stool floats and has a transit time of less than two days.

Note: Other supplements that can promote good elimination and prevent constipation include magnesium in combination with cascara sagrada, a gentle herb that stimulates bowel movements without cramping or addiction. This is a great alternative if the addition of fiber fails to remedy the problem of a sluggish bowel. Blonde psyllium seed husks contained in laxatives like Metamucil also lower cholesterol while treating constipation.

Control Your Sugar Intake: The Insulin Factor

Our diets are typically full of refined, empty carbohydrates that are easily accessible and rapidly digested, resulting in an influx of calories accompanied by blood sugar and insulin surges, as well as subsequent carbohydrate cravings. The average American diet consists of 15–20 percent sugars. To make matters worse, our deplorably low intake of fiber permits these highly refined sugars to jet into the blood stream due to their quick digestion. When a sweet food is fatless, it also leaves the stomach more rapidly, resulting in a shorter period of satisfaction and a rapid rise in blood sugar and insulin.

Simply stated, most of us eat too much starchy, sugary and fiberless foods, use saturated or hydrogenated fats and fail to consume enough raw fruits, vegetables, whole grains and nuts. The consequences of American eating habits include an increase in adipose tissue or body fat and elevated insulin levels due to the constant influx of sugar into the blood. Diabetes and obesity have reached epidemic proportions in the United States. Why? First of all, the ratios between our carbohydrate, protein and fat consumption are off. Couple that with vitamin and mineral depletion, high stress, a lack of exercise, eating excess meat and the continual snacking of high calorie, low nutrient foods, and you have the perfect formula for obesity and illness.

Insulin is a hormone that converts glucose to glycogen for the storage form of sugar housed in the liver and allows cells to absorb glucose for fuel. One of the most powerful influences on appetite is blood sugar level. We know that the more we stabilize blood sugar and insulin levels, the more we can control carbohydrate cravings (that incessant sweet tooth). Many women find that the week before their period hits, these food cravings escalate. In his book, *The Zone,* Barry Sears addresses what happens when we reach for starchy or sweet snacks to satisfy our hunger. "In desperation, your brain tells you that bag of corn chips looks very inviting. While eating the corn chips or (Oreo cookies) does supply an immediate source of carbohydrates for the brain, it simply restarts the vicious circle of raised insulin and diminished glucagon [stored sugar]."

Insulin and Estrogen

While many women link blood sugar to diseases like diabetes or obesity, few of them know that insulin levels influence estrogen and vice versa. Lowering your blood sugar by staying away from sweet and starchy foods brings insulin levels down, which helps to modulate the estrogen effect. In fact, we now have scientific evidence that women with high insulin levels have a dramatically higher risk of developing breast cancer whether they're slender or overweight. The more refined carbohydrates or high glycemic foods you eat, the more insulin is secreted into the bloodstream. Insulin may not only contribute to the estrogen effect but may also stimulate the growth of estrogen-dependent cancers. In fact, a report in the *American Journal of Obstetrics and Gynecology* points out that synthetic hormones found in HRT have an adverse effect on insulin resistance.

Insulin resistance refers to a condition where the pancreas secretes enough insulin, but the cells do not respond to its presence. Therefore, high circulating insulin levels persist. Insulin resistance is a major contributor to heart disease, obesity, high blood pressure and related conditions. We're also convinced that the high glucose diet of many women who believe that a no fat, high carbohydrate food is a free food is a great contributor to the estrogen/progesterone imbalances linked to the myriad of dis-

EXCESS WEIGHT AND ESTROGEN CONCERNS

Carrying around excess weight can worsen estrogen-driven symptoms. You see, not only is body fat percentage related to breast cancer risk, it also participates in the production of estrogen. It has been speculated that one reason obese women have more symptoms after menopause is that they have more circulating estrogen. Fat reserves work to manufacture estrogen, which serves to complicate hormonal balances from adolescence to the postmenopausal years.

eases discussed in this book. According to an article in a 1991 issue of the *Journal of Reproductive Medicine*, the consumption of foods and beverages high in sugar is associated with the prevalence of PMS.

Eat more high quality protein and be wary of the carbohydrate load you may be heaping onto your endocrine system. Get a glycemic index, and stay away from high glycemic foods. The higher a food's glycemic value, the faster it converts to blood sugar. You'll be surprised to find that many of the complex carbohydrates you thought were desirable foods have a high glycemic rating. Moreover, several foods considered ideal for weight loss are high in sugar, which can easily convert to fat. Simply stated, choosing foods lower in glycemic value, balancing them out with proper ratios of proteins and good fats and exercising is the key to preventing carbohydrate-related maladies, including the estrogen effect. Remember that if you keep blood sugar and insulin levels under control, you can receive the following benefits:

- enhanced energy and stamina
- better mental focus
- better cholesterol profile
- reduced risk for high blood pressure
- reduced risk for cardiovascular disease
- reduced risk for breast cancer
- better estrogen balance
- reduced body fat

Remember that using artificial sweeteners to lower your glucose load is a subject that's filled with controversy. Personally, we recommend using stevia, a powerful herbal sweetener that is considered safer than aspartame or saccharine.

Overall Dietary Guidelines for Hormone Health

- Eat good fats in moderation, emphasizing omega-3 and omega-9 fats, and limit omega-6 fat intake.
- Eat plenty of cabbage, broccoli, Brussels sprouts and cauliflower.
- Eat foods rich in fiber and potassium such as beans, sprouts, whole grains, almonds, sunflower seed, lentils, split peas, parsley, blueberries, endive, oats, potatoes with skin, carrots and peaches.
- Eat insoluble fiber on a daily basis like wheat bran, oat bran and related products.
- Eat very little or no white flour or sugar. Use whole grains and high quality protein foods like soy.
- Avoid alcohol, soda pop, caffeine and tobacco.
- Try to use lean meats from animals that have not been hormonally supplemented.
- Use organic produce free of pesticides.

A Word on Supplementation

We are firm believers of taking certain supplements. In an ideal world, eating a well-balanced diet would provide us with all the nutrients we need. Unfortunately, many of us exist in worst case scenarios, and even those of us who really try may still find that our diets are nutrient-deprived. We don't believe the RDA was ever set up to deal with the nutrient-depleting effects of stress, pollution, caffeine, etc. For example, here are some recent findings that powerfully illustrate the value of certain kinds of supplementation.

- If women began to take good calcium supplements early enough, it is estimated that millions of dollars could be saved on medical care required to treat bone fractures of the elderly.
- Taking a general vitamin supplement can boost immune function in the elderly, making them less susceptible to infection.
- Using a vitamin and mineral supplement during pregnancy could cut two of the primary causes of infant death in half by reducing the incidence of severe birth defects and of low-birth weight infants.

The truth of the matter is that even if you are eating a well-balanced diet, you're probably among the 95 percent of Americans who are lacking in at least one major mineral. In addition, the problem of mineral-poor earth is rarely addressed. As far back as 1936, U.S. Senate Document No. 264 warned Americans that the soils used to grow fruits and vegetables were seriously deficient in minerals. Continuous cropping and pollution were robbing our soil of the minerals needed to sustain life. Today the situation has not improved. A report from the 1992 Earth Summit shows that our earth's soil is anemic. In North America, 85 percent of the minerals in farm and range soils have been depleted over the last 100 years.

While taking specific supplements is certainly warranted, pills cannot provide the body with the vast diversity of nutrients found in the whole food as Mother Nature intended. The following supplements, however, can make a big difference in the lives of women and are suggested to augment soy for optimal hormone balance. They have several other health benefits as well.

Vitamins and Minerals for Hormone Balance

Vitamin B-Complex

There is some evidence that the B-complex vitamins may protect against some of the dangerous effects of estradiol and estrone in the body. Moreover, estrogen imbalances have been linked to a vitamin B6 deficiency. Using B vitamins can also help to ease the symptoms of PMS and fight depression and stress.

Vitamin B6

Vitamin B6 specifically treats water retention and helps to fight mood swings that can occur during PMS or menopause. Health professionals recommend taking twenty to fifty milligrams daily.

Vitamin E

Tests with vitamin E dramatically support its use for hot flashes and other menopausal symptoms. In some tests, it also worked better than barbiturates to calm anxiety. While some controversial data surrounding the use of vitamin E and breast cancer exists, the overwhelming consensus is that this vitamin helps to prevent breast fibroids; reduces the risk of heart disease; and may help to ease hormonally-induced symptoms. We recommend 200–400 IU daily of natural-source vitamin E products.

Vitamin C with Bioflavonoids

Clinical studies of menopausal women found that using vitamin C with hesperidin (a bioflavonoid) relieved symptoms in 50 percent of ninety-four women who participated in the study. Leg cramps, bruising and hot flashes also significantly decreased. Interestingly, certain bioflavonoids actually resemble estradiol in their chemical structure. Five hundred to 1,000 milligrams daily is the recommended dosage.

Calcium and Magnesium

These two minerals help to calm anxiety by quieting the central nervous system. They also provide a buffer against bone loss, which threatens some women after menopause when the risk of osteoporosis increases due to an estrogen decline. One thousand five hundred milligrams of calcium and 1,000 milligrams of chelated magnesium are recommended daily.

Vitamin D

Many postmenopausal women have impaired synthesis of vitamin D, which inhibits the absorption of calcium. Doctors suggest taking 400–800 IU daily.

Other Natural Compounds for Hormonally Driven Symptoms

Gamma-Oryzanol

This compound is extracted from rice bran and can help to modulate hot flashes and other menopausal symptoms, as seen in case studies. Suggested dosage is twenty milligrams daily.

5-Hydroxy-Tryptophan

Studies have found that low blood levels of tryptophan and estrogen were found in women who suffered from depression during menopause. Moreover, the 5-hydroxy-tryptophan compound may also help promote more restful sleep, which can be impaired during menopause. An article in the *Journal of*

Psychiatry and Neuroscience stated that supplemental trypto-phan also reduced several symptoms of PMS including insomnia, irritability and carbohydrate cravings. Suggested dosage is 100–200 milligrams three times daily.

Hormone-Friendly Herbs

Black Cohosh Root

Black cohosh root has been proven to be such an effective phy-toestrogen for menopausal disorders and premenstrual complaints that it has received official recognition in Britain and Germany. Studies have shown that black cohosh root has endocrine activity similar to soy isoflavones, in that it can mimic estrogen. Antispasmodic and diuretic actions are other properties that con-tribute to the herb's usefulness for women. Black cohosh is used for hot flashes, vaginal dryness and even the depression associated with menopause. Two to four milligrams daily of the extract (also called *Cimicifuga racemosa*) are recommended. This herb should not be used by pregnant or nursing women or in large doses.

Dong Quai

There is no other herb used more widely in Chinese medicine for treatment of gynecological ailments than dong quai. Dong quai, also called the "female ginseng," helps to relieve a number of unpleasant symptoms associated with menopause. It is believed to have analgesic properties, which is probably due in part to its antispasmodic effect. Dong quai also boosts elimina-tion, has both antiestrogenic and mild estrogenic properties and supports the cardiovascular system—all very valuable actions for menopausal women.

Take one fourth teaspoon of an extract daily (or 500–1,000 mil-ligrams daily). This herb should not be used by pregnant or nursing women or by anyone with hemorrhagic disease. It should also be avoided during severe cases of influenza. Exposure to the sun while taking this herb has caused a rash or aggravated sunburn in some people.

Chaste Berry (Vitex)

This herb acts on the pituitary gland to normalize hormonal function. Clinical evidence bears out the traditional use of vitex in the treatment of PMS, menopausal complaints and even infertility. A team of German investigators conducted a controlled, double blind study to evaluate the efficacy and safety of a standardized vitex supplement in comparison with pyridoxine (vitamin B6) in 175 women with PMS. Vitex was associated with a considerably better alleviation of typical PMS complaints, such as breast tenderness, edema, tension, headache, constipation and depression. Use a standardized product that contains 0.5 agnuside and take 175–225 milligrams daily.

Licorice Root

Licorice root is used in about a third of all Chinese herbal formulas and is widely used for female disorders. Licorice root controls water retention, breast tenderness, carbohydrate cravings and hormone imbalances. It also helps decrease some of the symptoms associated with hormone fluctuation. Use only deglycyrrhizinated (DGL) licorice root products, and take 250–500 milligrams daily. This herb should be avoided by anyone with high blood pressure, heart arrhythmia, kidney disease, or anyone on digoxin-based drugs or digitalis, unless supervised by a physician. Taking licorice root for extended periods can raise blood pressure. Taking potassium supplements with licorice root is advised.

Saw Palmetto Berries

American Indians have used saw palmetto berries for hundreds of years. Today this herb has been scientifically and clinically proven effective for male and female genitourinary problems. One study has shown it to be many times more effective than prescription anti-inflammatory medication in the treatment of pelvic congestion associated with menstrual dysfunction. Saw palmetto's popularity today centers around its use for prostate health. It offers considerable health benefits for women as well. Use fat-soluble standardized extracts that contain 85–95 percent fatty acids and sterols, and take 160 milligrams twice daily. Saw palmetto is considered safe and nontoxic.

Gotu Kola, Ginkgo Biloba and St. John's Wort

These herbs help to boost brain function and fight the anxiety, depression or lack of focus that can accompany PMS or menopause. Take as directed using standardized products or guaranteed potency products.

The Profound Value of Exercise

The value of regular exercise for women of all ages cannot be overemphasized. We've heard women profess on more than one occasion that exercising has preserved their physical well being as well as saved their sanity. Exercising can minimize the hormonally induced miseries that characterize menopause and can help ease crampy periods and the stress created by the ebb and flow of hormones during the menstrual cycle.

Clinical studies have found that hot flashes are half as common in women who engage in regular physical activity. Additionally, entering menopause with strong bones and toned muscles can enable the body to withstand menopausal physiological changes. Burning calories also helps to maintain ideal body weight, which may become more difficult with each passing year.

Carrying extra weight can also contribute to hormonal imbalances. Fat cells make estrogen, and it's usually not the good kind.

On the other hand, if a woman is too thin, she may experience even more estrogen depletion than normal during menopause, possibly making her symptoms worse than normal.

Exercising regularly is also considered by many experts to be the most significant weapon against the negative psychological symptoms that often characterize PMS and menopause. Engaging in some sort of aerobic workout (i.e., brisk walking, jogging or biking) three to five times a week for thirty-five to forty-five minutes is recommended. Working out with weights also builds muscle mass and helps prevent osteoporosis by maintaining bone density.

Moderate Exercise Can Be Effective

The key to successful exercising is to start slowly and to gradually build up. Choose the time of the day that feels the most natural to plan a simple regimen. While early morning may be the ideal time, make sure you're a morning person, or you will inevitably fail. You can use music to enhance your exercise routine. Music can motivate and energize your body so you move faster for longer periods of time.

Try to walk more. Walk around the block after work or walk a dog. Walk where and when it's safe, and walk consistently. Brisk walking is especially good. If you walk briskly for even ten minutes a day, you can expect to feel a considerable mental lift, and you will probably want to walk for longer periods of time. Begin where you feel comfortable and work up from there. Remember that some exercise is infinitely better than none. You should keep your goals realistic, or you'll stop altogether. If going outside is not an option, then use a treadmill, a stair-climber or go to an indoor track. We want to stress that even if you stay at your initial level and never progress to more strenuous workouts, that is perfectly acceptable. Ideally, all of us should at least be walking for thirty minutes at a brisk pace three to five times a week.

Exercise Formula

- Perform weight bearing exercises for thirty minutes three times a week: jogging, using a stair-climber or a treadmill, or walking (forty-five to ninety minutes, three times a week).
- Perform upper body strengthening exercises three times a week.
- Keep your exercise routine simple and practical; start slowly and build from there.
- Check with your doctor before you begin any exercise program.

Exercise and Stress

Understandably, if you are experiencing high stress, exercising is the last thing you feel like doing. However, releasing stress through exercise is highly recommended for its variety of beneficial effects, and more and more research supports the fact that exercise is a powerful therapy against the damaging effects of stress. Frequently, when we feel stressed out, we want to withdraw not only socially but physically as well. Did you know that some health care experts believe that becoming too sedentary creates stress itself? Numerous studies have discovered that breaking out of a lethargic life style results in more positive thoughts. Even seemingly minor, low impact exercise like walking around the block can release tension and can create desirable neurochemical changes in the brain.

The psychological benefits of regular exercise cannot be overemphasized, and all kinds of exercise can help to alleviate nervous tension. For this reason, you need to select the type of exercise that you will like and will do on a regular basis. Brisk walking is excellent and may be the perfect form of exercise. In addition, while you're walking, you can meditate, unraveling some of that stress. Exercise can naturally accomplish what drugs try to do—namely, elevate the brain amines that give us a sense of well being.

Most of us are aware of studies that show how endorphins in the brain are released after a certain amount of sustained exer-

THE MIND/BODY/SPIRIT CONNECTION

Someone once said, "Health is a state of complete physical, mental and social well-being, and not merely the absence of disease or infirmity." Stress is the great destroyer of life and needs the same aggressive therapy a physician would recommend for any serious disease. If you can't cut down on the stressors in your life, then try relaxation, workouts or even meditation. Dr. Herbert Benson, a cardiologist trained at Harvard University and author of *The Relaxation Response*, proved through his research that people who meditated for fifteen to twenty minutes per day reacted differently to stress. While it may be true that under stressful conditions their blood pressure would rise, it would only stay elevated for twenty or thirty minutes rather than for hours at a time. The effects of stress were markedly reduced for people who meditated regularly. If you can learn to incorporate this simple relaxation enhancer into your daily routine, you will experience profound changes in your outlook and in the way you handle stress.

cise and that these endorphins create a feeling of invigoration. It is also true that aerobic exercise causes norepinephrine to be released in brain cells, which helps to elevate mood. Exercise also raises the oxygen levels of cells, which can impact how much physical and mental energy we generate. When we breathe deeply, we expedite the removal of carbon dioxide and other waste products from our systems.

Exercise can be a marvelous release and can promote better relaxation and sleep. In light of its connection to the biochemical makeup of the brain, exercise can be an effective tool for alleviating and managing stress. Learning to walk briskly every day or to jog at a moderate pace not only eases stress but provides a whole host of physical benefits as well. Vigorous exercise can help relieve insomnia, promote good appetite and alleviate anxiety. It's also very inexpensive and helps to control weight and create fitness.

Spiritual Nourishment

Keep in mind also that regardless of your religious persuasion, drawing on the powers of heaven can help to enhance all facets of our health. One study called "The Efficacy of Prayer" by P.J. Collipp, M.D., suggested that prayer does indeed have value in the treatment of disease. Dr. Collipp states, "Among the plethora of modern drugs, and the increasing ingenuity of our surgeons, it seems inappropriate that our medical literature contains so few studies on our oldest and, who knows, perhaps most successful form of therapy [prayer]." Eric Fromm has said, "In addition to faith, we must possess courage, the willingness to take a risk, even to experience pain and disappointment." As humans, we often overlook some of the most powerful healing tools at our disposal. One of these tools is faith. Studies on this subject support the power of faith and prayer to greatly enhance the ability of an individual to recover from alcoholism, to stop smoking, to reduce blood pressure, to discourage depression or to improve the quality of life for cancer patients. Simply stated, our spiritual pulse can greatly affect our human condition.

Afterword

In all the years in which we have had the opportunity to research and use natural medicinal compounds, soy isoflavones stand out as truly remarkable phytonutrients. As we alluded to earlier, we are both surprised and concerned that the majority of our fellow physicians are not recommending soy's benefits to both their male and female patients. Women in our culture live in fear of diseases like breast cancer, deal with horrific hormonally-related disorders such as PMS, are prone to heart disease, find menopause difficult and believe that estrogen replacement therapy is their only option. Using soy foods on a regular basis, coupled with some of the other suggestions discussed in this chapter, may do more to help women manage these estrogen-related maladies than any other single dietary or pharmaceutical intervention. Learning to like soy foods is certainly a small thing compared to the potential health benefits this food offers us all. We can assure you that we have become soy-conscious and that we are actively spreading the word.

chapter 14

How to Become "Soy Savvy"

"A man's health can be judged by which he takes two at a time—pills or stairs."

JOAN WELSH

A Primer on Soy Protein

As we mentioned before, soy protein is a complete protein, which means that it contains all essential amino acids necessary for the building and maintenance of human body tissues. The body cannot manufacture essential fatty acids. They must be consumed in the diet or as supplements. The issue of whether soy can be considered a source of sulfur-containing amino acids called cystine and methionine depends on your definition of the word "source." Soy has some but not much of these two amino acids. Remember, however, that cystine is not an essential amino acid.

Based on new methods of rating protein designed by the Food and Drug Administration (FDA) and the World Health Organization (WHO), soy was given a score of one, which is the highest possible rating. Soy protein has now been elevated to a status equal to that of animal protein in its quality. Most people know that tofu is high in protein; however, not all soy foods are high in protein. Soy protein products come in three basic categories: isolated soy protein, soy concentrates and soy flours/grits. These forms of soy can be purchased and added to other foods. If you are trying to cut down on your meat consumption, you can add any of these forms of soy to ground beef as extenders.

Nix the Raw Soybean

Keep in mind that soybeans should not be eaten raw—they are unappealing and virtually impossible to eat in their raw state. There are good reasons why the raw bean is so inedible. The protease inhibitors found in the raw beans can actually inhibit protein breakdown in the body. Heating soy helps to counteract this effect. The phytic acid found in unprocessed soybeans may also compromise the body's ability to absorb minerals like calcium and iron, although some health experts consider the effect of this property negligible.

Isolated Soy Protein

Isolated soy protein (ISP) is the most refined form of soy protein and is frequently used in various meat products. It usually has a 92 percent protein content and comes in powders, granules and structured fibers. Isolated soy protein can also be used in very small amounts along with textured soy concentrate to help maintain juices during cooking. ISP has the appearance and texture of real meat and can actually enhance a food product's ability to withstand microwaving, freezing, thawing, etc. ISP will retain its isoflavone content if it has been processed with water rather than alcohol. It is considered a complete protein and is equivalent in protein quality to milk, meat or eggs, but it contains no cholesterol or saturated fats inherent to animal sources of protein and offers the body so many of the same benefits.

Textured Soy Protein

Textured soy protein (TSP) is made from textured soy flour and has a 70 percent protein content. Also referred to as textured vegetable protein (TVP), it was one of the first forms of soy protein to hit the market. It is available in dried granules, flakes and small chunks. When granules of TSP are rehydrated, the food resembles ground beef in its appearance and texture.

Soy Protein Concentrates

Soy protein concentrates are soy products that are the result of new processing technologies and are usually made from defatted soy flakes. Soy concentrates usually contain a 70 percent protein content. They have the ability to take on the flavor of foods they are added to and can improve the general quality of meat products due to their ability to retain moisture and flavor through a number of cooking processes. The two basic types of soy concentrates include textured soy concentrates and functional soy concentrates.

Textured Soy Concentrates

These come in flakes, small chunks or granules. Textured soy concentrates help to maintain the texture of foods when mixed with liquid and are commonly added to ground beef. Textured soy concentrates can give meat substitutes their meat-like texture and can preserve this texture through cooking, freezing or thawing.

Functional Soy Concentrates

These fine soy powders give a food product its firmness and moisture control. Just a little of this concentrate can make various food products juicier. These concentrates are often combined with textured soy concentrates to create a moist, meaty food.

Soy Flour and Soy Grits

Soy flours and grits comprise the least refined forms of soy protein. Soy grits resemble ground beef and have been used as texturizers in chili, spaghetti sauces, soups and stews. If soy flour is textured, it can also be used as a meat substitute. Soy technicians continually work to improve the consistency of soy flour so that it can be even more versatile.

Tofu

Tofu is a marvelous and exceptionally versatile food that is formed when hot soy milk is curdled, hence its designation as soybean curd. It is naturally low in saturated fat and contains no cholesterol. Its unique custard-like texture makes it perfect for all sorts of applications and because of its absorbency, it can take on the flavor of other foods it is mixed with. Tofu's soft consistency makes it an ideal protein source for children and elderly people, who may prefer foods that are easy to chew, especially since both groups can easily become protein deficient. Tofu can be pureed with fruits or vegetables in baby foods. There are generally four categories of tofu, and each one differs in firmness and nutrient content.

Extra-firm tofu: This type of tofu has less water content, making it quite firm. This type of tofu is ideal for slicing, dicing, frying and broiling. Typically, extra-firm tofu will also have a higher fat and protein content than other forms. You can successfully freeze and thaw extra-firm tofu, and you can also serve it as a meat substitute in soups, stews, casseroles, lasagna and many other dishes.

Firm tofu: Though not quite as dense as extra firm tofu, firm tofu can still be sliced or diced quite easily. Chefs like to use firm

SOY FOOD	PROTEIN
Miso	11.8 g
Natto	17.7 g
Okara	3.2 g
Soy flour (defatted)	47.0 g
Soy flour (full-fat, raw)	34.5 g
Soy flour (full-fat, roasted)	34.8 g
Soy flour (low-fat)	46.5 g
Soy milk	2.8 g
Soy protein concentrate	58.1 g
Soy protein isolate	80.7 g
Soy sauce (tamari)	10.5 g
Soybeans (cooked, boiled)	16.6 g
Soybeans (dry roasted)	39.6 g
Soybeans (raw)	36.5 g
Soymeal (defatted)	45.0 g
Tempeh	19.0 g
Tofu (raw, firm)	15.8 g
Tofu (raw, regular)	8.1 g

Table 1: *Protein content of various soy products (per 100 g).*

tofu in desserts and creamy dressings. In addition, it can also be used as a cheese substitute in recipes that call for cottage cheese, ricotta, soft cheese spreads or cream cheese.

Soft tofu: This type of tofu is quite difficult to slice and is better suited for blending into dips, dressings and sauces. It can be used as an egg substitute or to replace sour cream or yogurt. Soft tofu has less protein and fat than other forms.

Silken tofu: This tofu has a much more refined consistency and comes in extra firm, firm and soft. Silken tofu has all the same applications as other forms of tofu and is usually packaged in shelf-stable boxes.

Tofu contains nine amino acids and is a high-quality source of vegetable protein. It also contains calcium and is sometimes fortified with additional calcium, which is used as part of the curdling process. Check your tofu label for calcium content. Tofu is also a good source of isoflavones. Remember to rinse the tofu thoroughly with water.

Storing Tofu

The majority of tofu products have been pasteurized, and according to U.S. Food and Drug Administration (FDA) regulations, these products must be kept cold during distribution. Aseptically packaged tofu can be purchased and requires no refrigeration until opened. Always check the expiration date on the tofu package. Tofu can be stored for up to one week in the refrigerator if it is covered with water that is changed daily. Water keeps the tofu hydrated and prevents it from absorbing flavors or smells from adjacent foods. Aseptically packaged tofu needs to be eaten within two or three days. All types of tofu can be frozen for up to six months. Frozen tofu that has been defrosted will be chewier in its texture.

Soy Flour

Soy flour is made from grinding roasted soybeans into a fine powder. Rich in high-quality protein and other nutrients, soy flour can add an appealing texture and flavor to a number of food products. Soy flour can be purchased in either its natural full-fat form or a defatted variety. Full-fat soy flour contains all the natural oils found in the soybean. In defatted soy flour, a special process removes these oils. Both kinds of soy flour contain protein; however, the defatted from has a higher protein concentration. Both kinds of flour should be stored in the refrigerator or the freezer and should be stirred before using. Soy flour can be added directly to foods or recipes, or it can be toasted in a dry frying pan over moderate heat to bring out a nuttier flavor. Because soy flour tends to brown more rapidly, you may have to lower the baking temperature or decrease baking time for certain foods.

American cooks aren't used to using soy flour; however, it is found in numerous commercially prepared foods such as pies, pastries, candies, rolls, pancake mixes and doughnuts. Like wheat flour, soy flour can be used to thicken gravies and cream sauces. Using soy flour is an excellent way to add protein to foods normally high in carbohydrates only. Soy flour also boosts the shelf life of foods and helps reduce the fat absorption of doughs and batters. It also contributes to a more moist and tender consistency of foods.

Soy flour does not contain gluten; therefore, it cannot be used alone for breads. Add two to three tablespoons of soy flour to any yeast bread dough recipe for extra moistness. For nonyeast breads, substitute one fourth the amount of total flour with soy flour. Soy flour has also been used to replace eggs in recipes. One tablespoon of soy flour and one tablespoon of water is equivalent to one egg.

SOY FLOUR	FULL-FAT, ROASTED	DEFATTED
Calories	441	329
Protein (g)	34.80	47.00
Fat (g)	21.90	1.20
Carbohydrate (g)	33.70	38.40
Fiber (g)	2.20	4.30
Calcium (mg)	188.00	241.00
Iron (mg)	5.80	9.20
Zinc (mg)	3.50	2.40
Thiamine (B1)(mg)	41.00	7.00
Riboflavin (mg)	94.00	25.00
Niacin (mg)	3.29	2.61

Table 2: Nutrients in soy flour per 3.5 ounces (by weight).

Source: Composition of Foods: Legume and Legume Products. United States Department of Agriculture, Human Nutrition Information Service, Agriculture Handbook, Number 8–16. Revised, December 1986.

Soybean Oil

Soybean oil is one of the world's most commonly used oils. In the United States alone, soybean oil makes up almost 80 percent of edible oil consumption. The majority of all margarines and shortenings contain soybean oil. It also is commonly used in mayonnaise, salad dressings, frozen foods, imitation dairy and meat products and commercially baked goods. It is bland in flavor, which can be an advantage in some foods because it can assume any flavor. Soybean oil, if hydrogenated, is not recommended for everyday use. Soybean oil that is not hydrogenated has a high polyunsaturated oil content, although it does contain some monounsaturated fats and linolenic acid as well, which belong to the family of the omega-3 fats. Soybean oil has 61 percent polyunsaturated fat and 24 percent monounsaturated fat. Monounsaturated oils and fish oil are now considered our best bet when it comes to healthy fats, especially for women.

Unhydrogenated soybean oil is certainly not a bad choice of oils, but it should be used in moderation and in combination with the other good fats we discussed earlier. In addition, keep in mind that soybean oil is not a good source of isoflavones.

Soy Milk

Soy milk is gaining popularity as a delicious and versatile beverage that is particularly appealing for anyone who is lactose-intolerant because it is lactose and casein-free. Soy milk has a smooth, creamy texture and just a hint of sweetness that makes it the perfect base for shakes and smoothies. In fact, using soy milk is one of the easiest ways to add soy to your daily diet. It can be used like cow's milk.

Soy milk is made by grinding hulled soybeans and then cooking them with water. The water is eventually filtered and sweetened. Soy milk usually comes in ready-to-drink containers such as aseptic packages. You can buy fat-free soy milk, low-fat soy milk, fortified soy milk and soy-and-rice milk blends. You can find soy milk in health food stores or at the grocery near the evaporated or dry milk aisles. Packaged soy milk does not have to be refrigerated until after it is opened, after which it will keep fresh for approximately five days. You can also find soy milk in plastic containers much like cow's milk in the refrigerated dairy section. Powdered soy milk is also an option and should be stored in the refrigerator or freezer.

Powdered soy milk, once it is made, will need to be refrigerated and used within a week. Most soy milk powders are made from a combination of tofu powder and soy protein isolate with added sweeteners. Chocolate, strawberry, carob and vanilla prepared soy milks are also available. Sweetening agents used in soy milk include: barely malt, raw cane crystals and brown rice syrup. The taste of soy milk can vary from brand to brand, so if you don't like one, try another. At this writing, soy milk is still quite pricey, at an average of close to two dollars a liter. Prices will inevitably come down as soy foods gain popularity. You can also make your own soy milk to cut down on costs (refer to the recipe below).

Soy milk contains protein, thiamine, iron, phosphorous, copper, potassium and magnesium. It contains very little sodium. Depending on the product, some brands of soy milk are fortified with calcium, vitamin D and vitamin B12. Unlike cow's milk, soy milk is low in saturated fat and is cholesterol free. Standard nutrient tables list one cup of soy milk as providing 79 calories, 4.6 grams of fat (52 percent of calories), 6.6 grams of protein, 130 milligrams of sodium and 2 grams of fiber. The addition of certain sweeteners, vitamins, minerals and other ingredients can considerably change this profile. Keep in mind that unfortified soy milk contains approximately 40 milligrams of calcium per cup. Fortified products range in calcium counts from 200 to 400 milligrams per cup. Most soy milk powders are mixed with water and contain 0–8 grams of fat and 6–8 grams of protein. Remember that if you want to replace cow's milk with soy milk, you will need to purchase products fortified with calcium and vitamin D.

Homemade Soy Milk

1 cup soybeans
1/2 teaspoon and 1/8 teaspoon baking soda
2 ounces (60 grams) sugar, or to taste
pinch (2 grams) salt

Use clean, good quality soybeans that are free from dirt. Remove cracked, damaged and discolored soybeans.

Bring four cups water to a vigorous boil and add one half teaspoon baking soda. Drop one cup soybeans directly into the rapidly boiling water and blanch for five minutes. Drain and rinse with hot water.

Grind the blanched soybeans with seven cups very hot water (near boiling) for three minutes using a blender set at high speed. Filter the soybean mixture (soy slurry) by pouring it through cheese cloth. After the soy slurry in the cheese cloth has cooled to a safe temperature (to avoid burning), hand-squeeze the cheese cloth to extract as much soy milk as possible.

Add salt and sugar. Flavors (vanilla, chocolate, or others) may be added according to preference. Simmer (cook near boiling) for twenty minutes. Stir frequently to avoid burning.

Serve hot or cold. Refrigerate remainder, or if possible, consume by the end of the day. Makes about six cups of soy milk.

From Karl Weingartner at the University of Illinois

Soy Nut Butter

Soy nut butter is made from roasted soybeans commonly combined with soybean oil, corn syrup, soy protein isolate, evaporated cane juice, salt and mono- and diglycerides from vegetable sources. It is lower in fat and higher in nutrients than peanut butter and commonly comes in plastic jars, tubs or glass containers. Soy nut butter is usually only available in health food stores and is still rather expensive. Prices range from $3.69 to $5.59 for a jar.

Soy nut butter, like peanut butter, does not need refrigeration, even after it is opened. In fact, refrigerating soy nut butter will make it too difficult to spread. Also, oil separation is natural in soy nut butter, so it requires stirring before using.

Soy nut butter is an excellent source of soy protein and also contains omega-3 and omega-6 fatty acids. It has less fat than regular peanut butter. Isoflavone content will vary with each product, and while most manufacturers do not list it, soy nut butter should supply a significant amount of isoflavones. Thirty to forty milligrams of isoflavones are typically contained in a two-tablespoon serving.

Each two-tablespoon serving of soy nut butter generally contains 170 calories, 11 grams fat, 1.5 grams saturated fat, 6 grams polyunsaturated fat, 2.5 grams monounsaturated fat, 0 milligrams cholesterol, 170 milligrams sodium, 1 gram fiber, 10 grams carbohydrate, 8 grams protein and maybe a very small amount of iron and calcium.

Miso

Miso is nothing more than fermented soybean paste. It has a distinctive, full-bodied and salty flavor, which makes it the perfect addition to soups, stews, sauces, dressings, marinades and dips. Miso is made from combining soybeans, rice or barley; salt and water. The mixture is then fermented for up to three years. Miso comes in a variety of colors ranging from a rich brown to a mild yellow. Its color reflects the ratio of soybeans to rice, the amount of salt and the fermentation time. As would be expected, darker miso has a stronger flavor. You can buy miso in dehydrated or paste form. Typically, dehydrated miso has a shelf-life of approximately one year and should be stored in a cool, dry place. Miso paste should be kept in the fridge and will usually last for about six months. Miso comes in eight-ounce or one-pound tubs and in all kinds of varieties. It is usually salty but can also be sweet. Due to its high salt content, miso should be used sparingly to avoid an overload of sodium.

Miso is considered a good source of high-quality protein and carbohydrates that is low in calories and fat. Miso does have high salt content, so it should be used in small amounts for flavoring, as much as you would use salt.

Tempeh

Tempeh is a cultured cake made from soybeans that is often used as a meat substitute and is typically sold in eight-ounce patties. It has a chewy consistency that holds together so it can be easily grilled, deep-fried, baked, grated or microwaved and topped with all kinds of sauces. Tempeh is made by cooking and hulling soybeans and subsequently exposing them to a culture starter (much like sourdough bread is). The soybeans can also be combined with rice or barley. The mixture is then incubated at a certain temperature, which causes the beans to bind together into slabs that are eventually cut into smaller blocks and packaged. The fermentation process gives tempeh its nutty taste and may increase the availability of the soybean's isoflavones. Frozen, packaged tempeh will stay well preserved for up to a year or more. After it is thawed, it will store in the fridge for about a month. Tempeh cakes can appear to be whitish in color, which is perfectly normal; however, any green coloring indicates the presence of mold and means the product should not be used.

Tempeh is considered an excellent source of high-quality protein and is low in saturated fat. It also has the advantage of a higher fiber content and can significantly contribute to our adult daily requirement for dietary fiber. In addition, tempeh supplies the body with calcium, B vitamins and iron and contains no cholesterol. The fermentation of soybeans may actually make isoflavones more bioavailable because the mold used to make tempeh actually breaks into the section of the soybean where the majority of genistein is found. Fermentation also boosts riboflavin, niacin and folate compounds, while simultaneously lowering fat and thiamin counts. The nutritional value of tempeh will vary with each product, although a two-ounce serving of tempeh typically contains 113 calories, 4 grams of fat (nearly all of it unsaturated) and 11 grams of protein.

Whole Soybeans

Soybeans come in two varieties: dry soybeans and green vegetable soybeans, which undergo different harvesting methods. Dry soybeans are harvested when considered fully grown and dry. They are usually a light tan or yellow color and, if packaged in airtight containers, can last for indefinite periods of time like other hard beans. Green vegetable soybeans (also called edamame) are harvested just before they mature and resemble a pea in both their size and color. Green vegetable soybeans provide chefs with a versatile side dish or addition to salads and soups. Whole soybeans can usually be found in the legume section of health food stores or can be ordered through catalogs. Depending on your location, green vegetable soybeans can be purchased fresh from some produce or Asian markets, although they are more readily found frozen. Fresh green soybeans won't last much longer than two or three days and should be refrigerated. Frozen beans can last up to several months. Like any hard bean, the whole dry soybean takes a long time to cook and should be presoaked.

One-half cup of dry soybeans contains 149 calories, 7.7 grams of fat and 14.3 grams of protein. One-half cup of green vegetable soybeans contains 60 calories, 2 grams of fat and 6 grams of protein. Whole soybeans also contain 87 milligrams of calcium, 46 micrograms of folic acid and 4.4 milligrams of iron, as well as more than 5 grams of dietary fiber per half cup cooked portion.

How to Use Dry Soybeans

Dry soy beans need to be soaked overnight. In a large pot, add six cups of water for each pound of dry beans. Soak overnight or for eight hours. You can shorten the soaking time by bringing the water and beans to a boil and cooking for ten minutes. Remove the pot from the heat, cover it and let stand for one hour. Before the final cooking process whether you slow or quick soak the beans, drain and rinse them, and then put the soaked beans in a large pot. Add six cups of fresh water for each pound of beans and bring to a boil. Do not salt. Reduce heat and simmer for about three hours, until beans are tender. Undercooked soybeans do not digest well and do not taste the way they should. A pressure cooker can significantly decrease cooking time. Canned soybeans are available but aren't nearly as delicious as home-cooked beans.

How to Prepare Green Vegetable Soybeans

Firmly press bean pods between the thumb and forefinger to force beans out of the pods. Place one pound of green soybeans in a sauce pan of boiling, salted water. Bring back to a boil, then reduce heat, cover and simmer ten to fifteen minutes, until beans are tender. Serve immediately.

Frozen green soybeans are also available and can be steamed and eaten with sweet pepper, garlic and sesame oil.

Note: Cooked soybeans can be frozen in two-cup portions in freeze-lock bags for easy access.

Reference Information

Alphabetical List of Soy Foods Taken from the U.S. Foods Directory

Edamame (Green Vegetable Soybeans): These large soybeans are harvested when the beans are still green and sweet tasting. Edamame can be served as a snack or a main vegetable dish after being boiled in slightly salted water for fifteen to twenty minutes. These soybeans are high in protein and fiber and contain no cholesterol. Edamame are more often found in Asian and natural food stores, shelled or still in the pod.

Haelan: Haelan is a fermented soy beverage supplement that is rich in some vitamins, minerals and amino acids. Haelan is made by condensing twenty-five pounds of soybeans into an eight-ounce bottle and then fermenting the soybeans with *Azotobacter vinelandii.*

Hydrolyzed Vegetable Protein (HVP): HVP is a protein obtained from any vegetable, including soybeans. The protein is broken down into amino acids by a chemical process called acid hydrolysis. HVP is a flavor enhancer that can be used in soups, broths, sauces, gravies, flavoring and spice blends, canned and frozen vegetables, meats and poultry.

Kinnoko Flour: A Japanese food made from grinding soybeans into a fine powder, kinnoko flour is used to make sweets such as cookies and certain candies.

Lecithin: Extracted from soybean oil, lecithin is used in food manufacturing as an emulsifier for products high in fats and oils. It also promotes stabilization, antioxidation, crystallization and spattering control. Powdered lecithins can be found in natural and health food stores.

Meat Alternatives (Meat Analogs): Meat alternatives made from soybeans contain soy protein or tofu and other ingredients mixed together to simulate various kinds of meat. These meat alternatives are sold as frozen, canned or dried foods. Usually, they can be used the same way as the foods they replace. With so many different meat alternatives available to consumers, the nutritional value of these foods varies considerably. Generally, they are lower in fat, but read the label to be certain. Meat alternatives made from soybeans are excellent sources of protein, iron and B vitamins.

Miso: Miso is a rich, salty condiment that characterizes the essence of Japanese cooking. The Japanese make miso soup and use it to flavor a variety of foods. A smooth paste, miso is made from soybeans and a grain such as rice, plus salt and a mold culture, and then aged in cedar vats for one to three years. Miso should be refrigerated. Use miso to flavor soups, sauces, dressings, marinades and pâtés.

Natto: Natto is made of fermented, cooked whole soybeans. Because the fermentation process breaks down the beans' complex proteins, natto is more easily digested than whole soybeans. It has a sticky, viscous coating with a cheesy texture. In Asian countries, natto traditionally is served as a topping for rice and miso soups and is used with vegetables. Natto can be found in Asian and natural food stores.

Nondairy Soy Frozen Dessert: Nondairy frozen desserts are made from soy milk or soy yogurt. Soy ice cream is one of the most popular desserts made from soybeans and can be found in natural food stores.

Okara: A soy fiber by-product of soy milk, okara can be added as fiber to baked products.

Soy Cheese: Soy cheese is made from soy milk. Its creamy texture makes it an easy substitute for sour cream or cream cheese, and it can be found in variety of flavors in natural food stores. Products made with soy cheese include soy pizza.

Soy Fiber (Okara, Soy Bran, Soy Isolate Fiber): There are three basic types of soy fiber: okara, soy bran and soy isolate fiber. All of these products are high-quality, inexpensive sources of dietary fiber. Okara is a pulp fiber by-product of soy milk. It has less protein than whole soybeans, but the protein remaining is of high quality. Okara tastes similar to coconut and can be baked or added as fiber to granola and cookies, as well as being made into sausage. Look for okara in natural food stores. Soy bran is made from the soy hull (the outer covering of the soybean), which is removed during initial processing. The hulls contain a fibrous material that can be extracted and then refined for use as a food ingredient. Soy isolate fiber, also known as structured protein fiber (SPF), is soy protein isolates in a fibrous form.

Soy Flour: Soy flour is made from roasted soybeans ground into a fine powder. There are three kinds of soy flour available: natural or full-fat, which contains the natural oils found in the soybean; defatted, which has the oils removed during processing; and lecithinated, which has had lecithin added to it.
All soy flour gives a protein boost to recipes. However, defatted soy flour is an even more concentrated source of protein than full-fat soy flour. Although used mainly by the food industry, soy flour can be found in natural foods stores and some supermarkets. Soy flour is gluten-free so yeast-raised breads made with soy flour

are denser in texture. Replace one fourth to one third the flour with soy flour in recipes for quick breads, cakes, cookies, etc.

Soy Grits: Soy grits are similar to soy flour except that the soybeans have been toasted and cracked into coarse pieces, rather than the fine powder of soy flour. Soy grits can be used as a substitute for flour in some recipes. High in protein, soy grits can be added to rice and other grains and cooked together.

Soy Protein Concentrate: Soy protein concentrate comes from defatted soy flakes. It contains about 70 percent protein, while retaining most of the bean's dietary fiber.

Soy Protein Isolates (Isolated Soy Protein): When protein is removed from defatted soy flakes, the result is soy protein isolates, the most highly refined soy protein. Containing 92 percent protein, soy protein isolates possess the greatest amount of protein of all soy products. They are a highly digestible source of amino acids (the building blocks of protein necessary for human growth and maintenance).

Soy Protein, Textured: Textured soy protein (TSP) usually refers to products made from textured soy flour (TSF), although the term can also be applied to textured soy protein concentrates and spun soy fiber. Running defatted soy flour through an extrusion makes TSF, which allows for many different forms and sizes. When hydrated, TSP has a chewy texture. It is widely used as a meat extender.

One of the more popular brands of TSP is made by Archer Daniels Midland Company, which owns the right to the product named Textured Vegetable Protein (TVP). TSP contains about 70 percent protein and retains most of the bean's dietary fiber. TSP is sold dried in granular and chunk style. It can be found in natural food stores and through mail-order catalogs.

Soy Sauce (Shoyu, Tamari, Teriyaki): Soy sauce is a dark brown liquid made from soybeans that have undergone a fermenting process. Soy sauces have a salty taste but are lower in sodium than traditional table salt. Specific types of soy sauce are shoyu, tamari and teriyaki. Shoyu is a blend of soybeans and wheat. Tamari is made only from soybeans and is a by-product of making miso. Teriyaki sauce can be thicker than other types of soy sauce and includes ingredients such as sugar, vinegar and spices.

Soybeans, Whole: As soybeans mature in the pod, they ripen into a hard, dry bean. Most soybeans are yellow; however, there are brown and black varieties. Whole soybeans (an excellent source of protein and dietary fiber) can be cooked and used in sauces, stews and soups. Whole soybeans that have been soaked can be roasted for snacks and can be purchased in natural food stores and some supermarkets. When grown without agricultural chemicals, they are referred to as organically grown.

Soy Yogurt: Soy yogurt is made from soy milk. Its creamy texture makes it an easy substitute for sour cream or cream cheese. Soy yogurt can be found in variety of flavors in natural food stores.

Soy Milk, Soy Beverages: Soybeans that are soaked, ground fine and strained produce a fluid called soy milk, which is a good substitute for cow's milk. Plain, unfortified soy milk is an excellent source of high quality protein and B vitamins. Soy milk is most commonly found in aseptic containers (nonrefrigerated, shelf stable) but also can be found in quart and half-gallon containers in the dairy case at the supermarket. Soy milk is also sold as a powder, which must be mixed with water.

Soy Nut Butter: Made from roasted, whole soy nuts, which are then crushed and blended with soy oil and other ingredients, soy nut butter has a slightly nutty taste, significantly less fat than peanut butter and many other nutritional benefits as well. Soy nut butter can be found in a few supermarkets or through mail-order companies.

Soy Nuts: Roasted soy nuts are whole soybeans that have been soaked in water and then baked until browned. Soy nuts can be found in a variety of flavors, including chocolate-covered. High in protein and isoflavones, soy nuts are similar in texture and flavor to peanuts. You can find roasted soy nuts in natural food stores and through mail-order catalogs.

Soy Oil: Soy oil is the natural oil extracted from whole soybeans. It is the most widely used oil in the United States, accounting for more than 75 percent of our total vegetable fat and oil intake. Oil sold in the grocery store under the generic name "vegetable oil" is usually 100 percent soy oil or a blend of soy oil and other oils. Read the label to make certain you're buying soybean oil. Soy oil is cholesterol-free and high in polyunsaturated fat. Soy oil also is used to make margarine and shortening.

Sprouts, Soy: Although not as popular as mung bean sprouts or alfalfa sprouts, soy sprouts (also called soybean sprouts) are an excellent source of nutrition, packed with protein and vitamin C. They can be sprouted in the same manner as other beans and seeds. Soy sprouts must be cooked quickly at low heat so they don't get mushy. They can also be used raw in salads or soups or in stir-fried, sautéed or baked dishes.

Tempeh: Tempeh, a traditional Indonesian food, is a chunky, tender soybean cake. Whole soybeans, sometimes mixed with another grain such as rice or millet, are fermented into a rich cake of soybeans with a smoky or nutty flavor. Tempeh can be marinated and grilled and added to soups, casseroles or chili. Tempeh can be found in Asian food stores.

Tofu & Tofu Products: Tofu, also known as soybean curd, is a soft cheese-like food made by curdling fresh hot soy milk with a coagulant. Tofu is a bland product that easily absorbs the flavors of other ingredients with which it is cooked. Tofu is rich in high-quality protein, B vitamins and low in sodium. Firm tofu is dense and solid and can be cubed and served in soups, stir-fried or grilled. Firm tofu is higher in protein, fat and calcium than other forms of tofu. Soft tofu is good for recipes that call for blended tofu. Silken tofu is a creamy product and can be used as a replacement for sour cream in many dip recipes. Several types of tofu can be found in supermarkets and natural health food stores. Tofu is also available as a powder.

Whipped Toppings, Soy-Based: Soy-based whipped toppings are similar to other nondairy whipped toppings, except that hydrogenated soy oil is used instead of other vegetable oils.

Yuba: Yuba is made by lifting and drying the thin layer formed on the surface of cooling hot soy milk. It has a high protein content and is commonly sold fresh, half-dried and dried. In the United States, dried yuba sheets (called dried bean curd, bean curd sheets, or bean curd skin) and u-shaped rolls (called bamboo yuba or bean curd sticks) can be found in Asian food stores.

Isoflavone Content of Soy Foods

Soy foods can vary more than a hundred-fold in their isoflavone content. Keep in mind that second generation soy foods, such as soy burgers and hot dogs, are made from soy products that have been processed to improve flavor and texture. These processing techniques can also remove the isoflavone content of the soy food. On a dry weight basis, raw soybeans contain between two and four milligrams of total isoflavones per gram. Soy foods like tofu, miso, tempeh and soy milk that are commonly consumed in Asian countries are rich sources of isoflavones and provide approximately thirty to forty milligrams per serving. One-half cup of soy flour contains approximately fifty milligrams of isoflavones. Remember that soy sauce and soybean oil do not contain isoflavones. Soy protein concentrates (less than

65 percent soy protein) may or may not contain isoflavones, depending on which processing technique was used. Keep in mind that the isoflavone count of most commonly used soy protein concentrates is very low. Soy flour and textured soy protein are rich in isoflavones. Soy protein isolate (less than 90 percent soy protein) contains less isoflavones than these products but still has significant amounts.

Preferred Sources of Isoflavones

All the soy foods in the following list are excellent sources of isoflavones, providing a range of thirty to fifty milligrams per serving:

1 ounce roasted soy nuts
1/2 cup soy flour
1/4 cup soy grits
1/2 cup textured soy protein, cooked
1/2 cup yellow, green, vegetable or black soybeans, cooked
1 cup regular soy milk
1/2 cup tempeh
1/2 cup tofu

When in doubt as to the isoflavone content of a particular soy food, your best bet is to call the consumer line listed on the product label and ask the manufacturer for content information.

Soy Food	Daidzein	Genistein	Total Isoflavones
9-grain bread	0.01	0.01	0.02
Alfalfa seeds, sprouted, raw	0.00	0.00	0.00
Alfalfa seeds, sprouted, raw, mixed with clover seeds, sprouted, raw	0.00	0.00	0.00
Bacon, meatless	2.80	6.90	12.10
Beans, black, mature, seeds, raw	0.00	0.00	0.00
Beans, great northern, mature seeds, raw	0.00	0.00	0.00
Beans, kidney, all types, mature seeds, cooked, boiled, without salt	0.00	0.00	0.00
Beans, kidney, all types, mat. seeds, raw	0.02	0.04	0.06
Beans, kidneys, red, mature seeds, cooked, boiled, without salt	0.00	0.00	0.00
Beans, kidney, red, mature seeds, raw	0.01	0.00	0.01
Beans, navy, mature seeds, raw	0.01	0.20	0.21
Beans, pink, mature seeds, raw	0.00	0.00	0.00
Beans, pinto, mature seeds, raw	0.01	0.26	0.27
Beans, red, mature seeds, raw	0.00	0.31	0.31
Beans, small white, mature seeds, raw	0.00	0.74	0.74
Beans, snap, green, cooked, boiled, drained, without salt	0.00	0.00	0.00
Beans, snap, green, raw	0.00	0.00	0.00
Broadbeans (fava beans), mature seeds, raw	0.02	0.00	0.03
Broadbeans, fried	0.00	1.29	1.29
Chickpeas (garb. beans, bengal gram), mature seeds, raw	0.04	0.06	0.10
Clover sprouts, raw	0.00	0.35	0.35
Country rye bread, Finland	0.00	0.00	0.00
Cowpeas, common (blackeyes, crowder, southern), mature seeds, raw	0.01	0.02	0.03
Crackers, crispbread, rye	0.01	0.01	0.01
Flax seed, raw	0.00	0.00	0.00
Frichick (meatless chicken nuggets), canned cooked	4.35	9.35	14.60
Frichick (meatless chicken nuggets), canned, raw	3.45	7.90	12.20

Table 3: USDA-Iowa State U. database of isoflavone content of foods–1999.

Soy Food	Daidzein	Genistein	Total Isoflavones
Green Giant Harvest Burger, Orgnl. Flvr., All Veg. Protein Patties, frozen	2.95	5.28	9.30
Green Giant Harvest Burger, Original Flavor, All Vegetable Protein Patties, frozen, prepared	2.58	4.68	8.22
Infant formula, Enfamil Next Step, powder, soy formula	7.23	14.75	25.00
Infant formula, Mead Johnson Gerber soy, with iron, powder	8.08	13.90	25.09
Infant formula, Mead Johnson, Prosobee, w/ iron, liqu. cnctr.	1.10	2.22	6.03
Infant formula, Mead Johnson, Prosobee, with iron, powder	7.05	14.94	24.94
Infant formula, Mead Johnson, Prosobee, with iron, ready-to-feed	1.71	2.18	3.89
Infant formula, Ross, Isomil, with iron, powder	6.03	12.23	24.53
Infant formula, Ross, Isomil, with iron, ready-to-feed	1.91	2.26	4.17
Infant formula, Wyeth-a Yerst, Nursoy, with iron, liquid concentrate	1.02	2.82	4.02
Infant formula, Wyeth-a Yerst, Nursoy, with iron, powder	5.70	13.55	26.00
Infant formula, Wyeth-a Yerst, Nursoy, with iron, ready-to-feed	0.75	1.60	2.63
Instant beverage, soy, powder	40.07	62.18	109.51
Kala chana, mature seeds, raw	0.00	0.64	0.64
Lapacho tea (Tecoma heptaphylla)	0.02	0.03	0.05
Lentils, mature seeds, raw	0.00	0.00	0.01
Lima beans, large, mature seeds, cooked, boiled, without salt	0.00	0.00	0.00
Lima beans, large, mature seeds, raw	0.02	0.01	0.03
Lima beans, thin seeded (baby), mature seeds, raw	0.00	0.00	0.00
Miso	16.13	24.56	42.55
Miso soup mix, dry	24.93	35.46	60.39

Table 3: (cont.) USDA-Iowa St. U. database of isoflavone content of foods–1999.

Soy Food	Daidzein	Genistein	Total Isoflavones
Mung beans, mature seeds, raw	0.01	0.18	0.19
Mungo beans, mature seeds, raw	0.01	0.01	0.03
Natto (soybeans, boiled and fermented)	21.85	29.04	58.93
Oil, canola and soybean	0.00	0.00	0.00
Oil, soybean, salad or cooking	0.00	0.00	0.00
Peanuts, all types, raw	0.03	0.24	0.26
Peas, split, mature seeds, raw	2.42	0.00	2.42
Pigeon peas (red gram), mat. seeds, raw	0.02	0.54	0.56
Snacks, granola bars, hard, plain	0.05	0.08	0.13
Soybean butter, full-fat, Worthington Foods, Inc.	0.22	0.30	0.57
Soy cheese, unspecified	11.24	20.08	31.32
Soy cheese, cheddar	1.80	2.25	7.15
Soy cheese, mozzarella	1.10	3.60	7.70
Soy cheese, parmesan	1.50	0.80	6.40
Soy drink	2.41	4.60	7.01
Soy fiber	18.80	21.68	44.43
Soy flour (textured)	59.62	78.90	148.61
Soy flour, defatted	57.47	71.21	131.19
Soy flour, full-fat, raw	71.19	96.83	177.89
Soy flour, full-fat roasted	99.27	98.75	198.95
Soy hot dog, frozen, unprepared	3.40	8.20	15.00
Soy meal, defatted, raw	57.47	68.35	125.82
Soy milk, fluid	4.45	6.06	9.65
Soy milk, iced	1.90	2.81	4.71
Soy milk skin or film (Foo jook or yuba), cooked	18.20	32.50	50.70
Soy milk skin or film (Foo jook or yuba), raw	79.88	104.80	193.88
Soy noodles, flat	0.90	3.70	8.50
Soy paste	15.03	15.21	31.52
Soy protein cnctr., aqueous washed	43.04	55.59	102.07
Soy protein concentrate, produced by alcohol extraction	6.83	5.33	12.47
Soy protein isolate	33.59	59.62	97.43
Soy sauce fr. hydrolyzed veg. protein	0.10	0.00	0.10

Table 3: (cont.) *USDA-Iowa St. U. database of isoflavone content of foods–1999.*

Soy Food	Daidzein	Genistein	Total Isoflavones
Soy sauce made from soy and wheat (shoyu)	0.93	0.82	1.64
Soy-based liquid formula for adults, Ross Enrich	0.14	0.40	0.54
Soy-based liquid formula for adults, Ross Glucerna	0.02	0.06	0.08
Soy-based liquid formula for adults, Ross Jevity Isotonic	0.03	0.31	0.34
Soybean chips	26.71	27.45	54.16
Soybean curd cheese	9.00	19.20	28.20
Soybean, curd, fermented	14.30	22.40	39.00
Soybeans, Brazil, raw	20.16	67.47	87.63
Soybeans, Japan, raw	34.52	64.78	118.51
Soybeans, Korea, raw	72.68	72.31	144.99
Soybeans, Taiwan, raw	28.21	31.54	59.75
Soybeans, flakes, defatted	36.97	85.69	125.82
Soybeans, flakes, full-fat	48.23	79.98	128.99
Soybeans, immature, cooked, boiled, drained, without salt	6.85	6.94	13.79
Soybeans, immature, seeds, raw	9.27	9.84	20.42
Soybeans, green, mature seeds, raw	67.79	72.51	151.17
Soybeans, mature cooked, boiled, without salt	26.95	27.71	54.66
Soybeans, mature seeds, dry roasted	52.04	65.88	128.35
Soybeans, mature seeds, raw (U.S., food quality)	46.64	73.76	128.35
Soybeans, mature seeds, raw, (U.S., commodity grade)	52.20	91.71	153.40
Soybeans, mature seeds, sprouted, raw	19.12	21.60	40.71
Soylinks, frozen, cooked, Morning Star breakfast	0.75	2.70	3.75
Soylinks, frozen, raw, Morning Star breakfast	1.18	2.45	3.93
Spices, fenugreek seed	0.01	0.01	0.02
Sunflower seed kernels, dried	0.00	0.00	0.00
Tea, green, Japan	0.01	0.04	0.05

Table 3: (cont.) *USDA-Iowa St. U. database of isoflavone content of foods–1999.*

Soy Food	Daidzein	Genistein	Total Isoflavones
Tea, jasmine, Twinings	0.01	0.03	0.04
Tempeh	17.59	24.85	43.52
Tempeh burger	6.40	19.60	29.00
Tempeh, cooked	19.25	31.55	53.00
Tofu, Mori-Nu, silken, firm	11.13	15.58	27.91
Tofu, dried-frozen (koyadofu, kori tofu, or tung tou-fu)	25.37	42.15	67.49
Tofu, Azumaya, extra firm, prepared with nigari	8.23	12.45	22.63
Tofu, Azumaya, firm, cooked	12.80	16.15	31.35
Tofu, firm, prepared with calcium sulfate and nigari	9.44	13.35	24.74
Tofu, fried (aburage)	17.83	28.00	48.35
Tofu, okara	5.39	6.48	13.51
Tofu, pressed (Tau kwa), raw	13.60	13.90	29.50
Tofu, raw, regular, prepared with calcium sulfate	9.02	13.60	23.61
Tofu, salted and fermented (fuyu)	14.29	16.38	33.17
Tofu, soft, VitaSoy-silken	8.59	20.65	29.24
Tofu, soft, prepared with calcium sulfate and nigari	11.99	18.23	31.10
Tofu, yogurt	5.70	9.40	16.30
USDA Commodity, beef patties with VPP, frozen, cooked	0.67	1.09	1.86
USDA Commodity, beef patties with VPP, frozen, raw	0.35	0.77	1.14
Worthington Foods, Loma Linda, Big Franks, meatless, franks, canned	1.00	2.05	3.35
Worthington Foods, Loma Linda, Big Franks, meatless, franks, canned, prepared	1.35	2.00	3.75

Table 3: (cont.) *USDA-Iowa St. U. database of isoflavone content of foods–1999.*

Questions and Answers About Soy

Q. *I rarely see genistein listed on a soy food label. How do I know how much is in a particular product?*
A. You usually won't know. The best you may hope for is to see a total isoflavone count, which includes genistein, daidzein and glycetein. Isoflavone content charts (like the one in this book) can give you the customary isoflavone counts of most soy foods, or you can call the consumer telephone number listed on a product label and ask the manufacturer directly.

Q. *I heard that soy has "antinutrients" that can block the absorption of calcium. Is this true?*
A. Soy does contain compounds called phytates and oxalates that can bind to minerals like calcium and iron, inhibiting their absorption. We do know that the calcium in soy is assimilated much the same way calcium in cow's milk is, suggesting that the body receives a good amount from foods like tofu and that the effect of phytates and oxalates is not significant.

Q. *Every time I turn around I see a different set of guidelines as to how much soy to eat. I'm afraid of not eating enough or eating too much soy. What is the best policy?*
A. As we've mentioned before, the Asian model should be our aim and moderation the best policy. We recommend eating no less than twenty-five and no more than sixty grams of soy daily. While the phytoestrogen content of soy foods varies considerably for each product, one or two servings of tofu, soybeans or soy milk a day is equivalent to the normal soy intake of Asian women, which includes approximately thirty-five milligrams of isoflavones. One cup of soybeans provides 300 milligrams of isoflavones.

Q. *I heard that giving a baby or child soy can cause them to experience premature puberty and early periods. Is this true?*

A. Soy-based infant formulas have been used in this country for decades without any indication that the early onset of menstruation or puberty has resulted from their use.

Q. *Can a woman take soy when she is taking HRT? Does it interfere with the action of synthetic estrogen?*

A. There is no evidence that eating soy foods in combination with HRT is a bad thing. On the contrary, we would highly recommend it due to soy's hormonally-protective properties.

Q. *Is soy milk an adequate source of calcium?*

A. It depends on whether you are substituting soy milk for cow's milk, in which case you will want to use soy milk that has been fortified with additional calcium and vitamin D. Unfortified soy milk contains four milligrams of calcium per 100 grams, which is not a high amount.

Q. *Can children drink soy milk?*

A. Unless your child is allergic to cow's milk, we suggest that you not give your child soy milk until your child is eighteen months old. Give your child full-fat varieties of cow's milk that are fortified. If your child is a vegetarian, give your child a B12 supplement as well.

Q. *Does full-fat soy milk contain more isoflavones?*

A. Fat has nothing to do with isoflavone content. Generally speaking, the more protein in the soy product, the higher the isoflavone content of that product. Isoflavone content can also be affected by different processing techniques.

Q. *Do high temperatures associated with frying and other forms of cooking destroy isoflavones?*

A. There is no indication that isoflavone structures are damaged by high cooking temperatures.

Q. *I learned about isoflavones from my neighbor who is taking them in supplement form, but I don't know how well isoflavone supplements work. Is taking supplements a good way to ensure that you are getting thirty-five milligrams of total isoflavones daily?*

A. The jury is still out on the safety and efficacy of isoflavone supplements. They may prove to be very valuable; however, at this point getting your isoflavones from soy foods is considered preferable.

chapter 15

Eating Soy and Loving It

"The discovery of a new dish does more for human happiness
than the discovery of a new star."
ANTHELME BRILLAT-SAVARIN

ONE OF THE most satisfying experiences we've had is to be introduced into the wonderful world of soy foods. Like so many of you, we were somewhat hesitant to give soy a chance because our food preferences so often reflect our cultural backgrounds. But let us just say, if you don't take the opportunity to include soy in your culinary creations, you'll be missing out on some of the most delightful taste sensations, not to mention the profound nutritive value that soy offers.

Because women so often control what their families eat, experimenting with soy foods and recipes, like the ones included here, can have an extraordinary impact on the health of spouses and children. If you're really serious about adding soy to your diet due to its hormonal hallmarks, you'll discover that it's easy to sneak soy into all kinds of foods that your family normally eats. It's just a matter of getting into the "soy habit" and keeping soy foods readily available.

The recipes included in this section are guaranteed to break even the most soy-resistant individuals. They come from the Indiana Soybean Board, the Soy Connection, Simply Soy and from other soy lovers. They are easy to prepare and absolutely delicious. Louise Tenney, noted herbalist and author of natural health books, uses tofu to make delicious side dishes to complement Sunday dinners and consistently hears "oooohs" and "aaahs" from her family members. Tofu is one of the most versatile foods you'll ever run across. Once you cook with it, you'll wonder how you ever got along without it. Even a soy novice will eventually find that eating at least one soy-based meal per day is not difficult. In fact, there are now a variety of large food production companies, like Kellogg's, Archer Daniels Midland, Arrowhead Mills and General Mills, that are taking serious strides in bringing soy to our tables in already prepared forms. So let's talk about some easy ways you can add soy into your everyday foods.

Easy Ways to Sneak Soy into Your Diet

Miso

- Use miso to add flavor to dressings, soups and sauces.
- Use miso as a substitute for anchovy paste, salt or soy sauce.
- For instant soup, mix one-quarter cup of miso in a quart of boiling water. Add chopped scallions and serve. A tablespoon of miso mixed into a cup of hot water makes an individual serving.

Tempeh

- Add cubes of tempeh to sloppy joe sauce, chili, stews, casseroles or soups.
- Grill marinated tempeh as a substitute to a meat entrée.

Tofu

- Add chunks of firm tofu to soups and stews.
- Blend crumbled tofu into meat loaves or taco meat.
- Mash tofu with cottage cheese and green onions to make a sandwich spread.
- Marinate tofu slices in barbecue or teriyaki sauce and cook on an outdoor grill as a side dish.
- Mix dried onion soup (or other flavors) into soft or silken tofu for a vegetable or chip dip.
- Blend silken tofu into sour cream by half.
- Blend silken tofu into pie fillings.
- Beat silken tofu into pudding recipes.
- Dip firm tofu into beaten egg and flour and fry in olive oil.
- Substitute silken tofu for half the cream in soups and related products.
- Use blended tofu for half the amount of mayonnaise, sour cream, cream cheese or ricotta cheese called for in recipes.
- Substitute blended soft tofu for sour cream in creamy salad dressing recipes.
- Beat an entire package of soft tofu into mashed potatoes. You won't taste the tofu, and the texture will be creamier than ever.
- Put cubes of tofu in any stir-fry recipe.
- Blend silken tofu into yogurt.

Textured Vegetable Protein (TVP)

- Add TVP to casseroles, meat, lasagna, manicotti, chili, pizza toppings or sloppy joes.
- Add TVP to stir-fry and taco salads.
- Add TVP to soups and stews.
- Try various veggie burgers made with TVP.

Soy Milk

- Use soy milk in batters for muffins, cookies, breads or cakes.
- Use soy milk over cereal for breakfast.

- Make milkshakes or smoothies using soy milk and fruit.
- Use soy milk (unflavored) to make cream sauces or creamed soups.
- Use soy milk in pancake and waffle mixes.
- Replace evaporated milk with soy milk in dessert recipes.
- Use soy milk in instant pudding recipes (use only half the amount of cow's milk).
- Use vanilla soy milk in cocoa recipes.
- Use soy milk instead of cream in your coffee.

Soy Flour

- Replace about one fourth of the flour in a cake, pancake or waffle batter, muffin or bread recipe with soy flour.
- Use soy flour to thicken gravies.

Soy Nut Butter

- Replace or partially substitute soy nut butter for peanut butter.
- Use soy nut butter on bagels and toast.
- Spread soy nut butter on apples or pears.
- Use soy nut butter as a cracker topper.
- Blend soy nut butter into shakes.
- Use soy nut butter in cookie recipes.

Soy Protein Powder

- Blend soy protein powder (containing soy protein isolate) with fruit juice and fresh fruit to make specialty drinks and shakes.
- Blend one to two tablespoons of soy protein powder into meat loaves, chili, soups and casseroles.

Whole Cooked Soybeans

- Use whole cooked soybeans to replace part of other beans called for in baked beans or barbecue bean recipes.
- Use whole cooked soybeans cold in salads.

Soy Nuts

- Add soy nuts to low-fat pretzels, crackers, Chex mix, etc. They have less than half the fat contained in peanuts and cashews.
- Grab a handful of roasted soy nuts for a snack.

Cholesterol-Containing Foods and Soy Substitutes

ice cream	vs.	tofu-based ice cream
cheeseburger	vs.	soy burger with soy cheese
ground beef	vs.	textured vegetable protein (TVP)
milk shakes	vs.	soy shakes made with soy milk
sour cream	vs.	seasoned creamed tofu
hot dog	vs.	soy dog
pork sausage	vs.	soy sausage
chicken/beef broth	vs.	miso soup
beef jerky	vs.	soy nuts

Recipes Guaranteed to Make You a Soy Lover

Specialty Drinks

Strawberry-Kiwi Smoothie

1 cup vanilla soy milk
1/2 large banana
2 tablespoons frozen lemonade concentrate (undiluted)
1/4 cup frozen strawberries
1 kiwi fruit, peeled

Place all ingredients in blender and puree until smooth. Serve immediately or refrigerate.

From Rita Elkins

Strawberry Banana Frosty

3 cups plain or vanilla soy milk
1 ripe banana
1 cup strawberries

Blend all ingredients in blender until smooth.

From the United Soy Board

Purple Power Shake

1 cup vanilla soy milk
1 cup firm tofu (about 6 ounces)
3/4 cup fresh or frozen, unthawed blueberries
1 teaspoon almond extract
2 scoops soy protein powder (1 scoop is about 3 tablespoons)

Place all ingredients in blender and mix on high until mixture is thoroughly blended and smooth and creamy. Serve immediately or refrigerate.

From the Indiana Soybean Board

Cranberry Raspberry Smoothie

1 cup vanilla soy milk
1/2 large banana
2 tablespoons frozen cranberry juice concentrate (undiluted)
1/4 cup frozen raspberries

Place all ingredients in blender and puree until smooth. Serve immediately or refrigerate. Makes 1 1/2 cups.

From the Indiana Soybean Board

Orange You Glad Smoothie

1 cup ice
2 cups vanilla soy milk
2 tablespoons soy protein powder
1/4 cup soft tofu
1 cup fresh orange juice
3/4 cup pure maple syrup
1 very ripe banana
1/2 teaspoon cinnamon or nutmeg (optional)

Blend on high until smooth and serve over ice. Sprinkle cinnamon or nutmeg on top if desired. Serve immediately.

From Rita Elkins

Breakfast Delights

Mushroom Scrambler (Egg-free)

1 pound firm tofu
2 teaspoons oil
2 cloves garlic, minced
4 cups sliced assorted mushrooms (brown, button and shiitake)
1/2 cup chopped green onions
1 teaspoon minced fresh rosemary
8 ounces egg substitute
1/2 cup grated Fontina cheese
salt and pepper to taste

Drain tofu and crumble into cottage cheese-sized pieces. Heat oil in large skillet and add tofu; cook over medium-high heat until tofu becomes light golden brown. Add garlic and cook three to four minutes more. Add mushrooms and continue to cook until mushrooms begin to brown, then add green onions and rosemary. Cook three to four minutes. Add egg substitute and cook just until liquid begins to set, then add cheese and salt and pepper to taste. Cook just until cheese begins to melt. Do not overcook.

From the Los Angeles Times, by Mayi Brady

Apple Pancakes

1 cup all-purpose flour
3 tablespoons sugar
1/2 teaspoon cinnamon
1/4 teaspoon nutmeg
1/8 teaspoon salt
2 teaspoons baking powder
3/4 cup soy milk
1 tablespoon soy flour

1 teaspoon vanilla extract
2 tablespoons margarine, melted and cooled
1 tart apple, peeled, cored and grated

Mix the sugar with cinnamon, nutmeg and salt. Blend sugar mixture with flour, soy flour and baking powder. In a separate bowl, whisk together the soy milk, vanilla extract and margarine. Pour liquid ingredients over the dry mixture and blend together. Fold in the apples. Pour 1/4 cupfuls of batter onto hot, nonstick griddle or pan. Cook for about two minutes on first side or until bubbles appear on surface. Flip and cook for another minute or until heated through. Serve topped with applesauce and maple syrup. Makes 12 pancakes.

From the United Soy Board

Banana-Oat Pancakes

1/2 cup rolled oats
1/2 cup unbleached flour
1/4 cup soy flour
1 tablespoon baking powder
1 1/2 cups plain soy milk
2 bananas, thinly sliced

In a large bowl, combine the rolled oats, unbleached flour, soy flour and baking powder. Add the soy milk, and blend with a few swift strokes. Fold in the banana slices. Pour 1/4 cupfuls of the batter onto a hot, nonstick griddle or pan. Cook for about two minutes or until bubbles appear on the surface. Flip the pancake and cook for another minute or until heated through. Serve the pancakes with maple syrup, fruit spread or applesauce. Makes 12 pancakes.

From the Indiana Soybean Board

Heart-Healthy Apricot Muffins

1 1/2 cups all-purpose flour
1/8 teaspoon salt
1/2 cup soy flour
1 egg
1/3 cup sugar
1/2 cup soy milk
1/2 cup water
1 tablespoon baking powder
1 tablespoon vegetable (soybean) oil
1 teaspoon ground cinnamon
1/2 cup crushed pineapple
1/2 cup dried apricots
1/4 teaspoon ground nutmeg

Combine flours, sugar, baking powder, spices and salt; mix well. Make a well in the center and add egg, soy milk, water, oil, pineapple and apricots; mix only until moistened. Spoon mixture into oiled muffin tins. Bake at 400°F for twelve to fifteen minutes or until wooden pick inserted near center comes out clean. Makes 12 muffins.

From the United Soy Board

Soy Pancakes

1 cup soy flour
2 3/4 cups all-purpose flour
3 tablespoons baking powder
3 tablespoons sugar
1 1/2 teaspoons salt
3 eggs
3 cups milk
6 tablespoons salad oil

Mix all ingredients together until moistened. (Add extra milk for thinner pancakes.) Spray griddle with a nonstick cooking spray. Preheat over to 350°F. Pour 1/2 cup of batter on griddle for each pancake. Makes 30 pancakes.

From Shirley Aufdenberg, Jackson, Mo., and Patricia Fornkohl, Cape Girardeau, Mo., and the Indiana Soybean Board

Muesli with Soy Nuts and Dried Fruit

1 1/2 cup low-fat granola (without raisins)
1 1/2 cup vanilla soy milk
1/2 cup raisins
1/2 cup dried cranberries
3/4 cup roasted soy nuts

Combine granola, soy milk and dried fruits in bowl or storage container. Cover and refrigerate several hours or overnight. Stir in soy nuts just before eating if crunchy nuts are desired; otherwise, add soy nuts along with other ingredients. The soy nuts will soften considerably. Makes 3 cups.

From the Indiana Soybean Board

Appetizers

Tofu Onion Dip

1/3 cup soft tofu
1/3 cup yogurt
4 tablespoons hot sauce
3 tablespoons red onion, diced
1 teaspoon dill weed
1/2 teaspoon garlic powder

236 / SOY SMART HEALTH

Cream hot sauce and a small amount of yogurt together until smooth. Blend in remaining yogurt and tofu, then add remaining ingredients. Refrigerate at least one hour before serving. Serve with chips or raw veggie sticks.

From the Maryland Soybean Board

Soybean and Roasted Red Pepper Sauce

This versatile sauce takes minutes to prepare. Use instead of tomato sauce for pizza. Drizzle on nachos or burritos. Use as a dip for baked tortilla chips. Spread a thin layer on hot cooked veggie burgers.

1 1/2 cup cooked soybeans
1 roasted red bell pepper (about 1/2 cup jarred roasted red bell pepper)
1/4 cup water or vegetable broth
2 tablespoons nutritional yeast flakes
1 tablespoon brown rice vinegar
1/2 teaspoon salt-free Onion Magic or onion powder
1/4 teaspoon salt (or to taste)
pinch of dried red pepper flakes, to taste (optional)

Blend all ingredients in a blender at high speed until smooth. Refrigerate until ready to use. To serve the sauce warm, heat gently in a saucepan or double boiler (do not simmer or boil). Makes about 2 cups.

From Vegging Out

Marinated Tempeh

You can make marinated tempeh ahead of time to have on hand for quick meal preparations. Ingredients can be varied to change the taste. Good additions include garlic powder, dry salad dressing mixes and flavored vinegars.

2 cups water or vegetable broth
2 tablespoons tamari or soy sauce
1 tablespoon brown rice vinegar or other mild vinegar
2 slices fresh ginger
2 cloves garlic, crushed
1 pound tempeh, cut into 2-ounce or 4-ounce pieces
1 teaspoon brown sugar
a dash of dry hot mustard

Combine all ingredients in a shallow dish, and chill for a minimum of one hour or overnight. Occasionally turn the tempeh chunks. Place ingredients in a saucepan, cover, and simmer for thirty minutes. Remove flavored tempeh and refrigerate. The remaining liquid can be used as a sauce to top vegetables or rice. Makes 4 to 8 servings.

Other ways to use marinated tempeh:

• Use marinated tempeh patties as vegetarian burgers.
• Use thinly sliced and chilled marinated tempeh in sandwiches and salads.
• Add cubed marinated tempeh to stir-fry dishes.
• Grated marinated tempeh adds flavor to casseroles, stews or soups.

From Rita Elkins

Mushroom Tempeh Pâté

This is a great party dish to make ahead of time. Serve it with poppy seed crackers or on slices of rye bread.

1 cup sliced fresh mushrooms (any variety)
1 small onion, minced
1 tablespoon olive oil
2 cloves garlic, minced
1 1/2 cup cooked or canned (drained) lima beans or white beans
8 ounces cooked marinated tempeh, crumbled

Sauté mushrooms and onion in olive oil for five minutes. Add garlic, and sauté three to five minutes more. Combine sautéed vegetables with beans and marinated tempeh in a food processor and blend until smooth. Transfer to a serving dish, and chill thoroughly. Serve garnished with fresh parsley. Makes just over 2 cups.

From Vegging Out

Soy Balls

4 cups cooked and coarsely ground soybeans
1 teaspoon garlic powder (or fresh minced)
1 teaspoon salt
1 teaspoon black pepper
green onion, onion, parsley (3 tablespoons each, chopped)
2 cups water
1 cup all-purpose flour
1 tablespoon baking powder
oil (for frying)

Mix all ingredients. Heat the oil and fry by teaspoonfuls.
From INTSOY, University of Illinois at Urbana-Champaign

Soups

Miso Soup

1 tablespoon olive or peanut oil
1 small onion, sliced
3 cups water
3 heaping tablespoons miso

2 tablespoons diced tofu
1 cup cooked noodles (Japanese ramen noodles work best)
chopped green onion

Sauté the onion in oil until tender. Add a small amount of the water to the onions, and add the miso to form a smooth paste. Add the rest of the water and the tofu, and cook on low heat for ten minutes. Add the cooked noodles, top with chopped green onions and serve. You can add any grain or vegetable you would like to the broth. Serve immediately. Makes 4 servings.

From Rita Elkins

Curried Carrot Soup

6 medium carrots, thinly sliced
2 cups vegetable stock
1 small onion, chopped
1/2 cup plain soy milk
2 teaspoons curry powder

Combine all ingredients except the soy milk and cook over medium heat until carrots are tender. Pour into a blender and puree until smooth. Stir in the soy milk. Cook over low heat until hot. Makes 4 servings.

From the Indiana Soybean Board

Potato and Pea Bisque

4 large unpeeled potatoes, cut into small cubes
1/2 large purple onion, finely chopped
2 cups water
1 teaspoon chicken bouillon powder or granules
1/2 teaspoon salt
1/4 teaspoon pepper
1 package frozen peas

1 cup plain soy milk
1/2 cup heavy cream
2 tablespoons flour
2 tablespoons butter

In a medium saucepan, combine the potatoes, onion, water, bouillon, salt and pepper. Bring to a boil, reduce heat and simmer until potatoes are tender, about fifteen to twenty minutes. Remove pan from heat and stir in the peas. Shake the flour in a covered container with the soy milk and cream, and add to the potato mixture. Cook slowly until thickened.

From Rita Elkins

Butternut Peanut Soup

Pair this rich soup with some good sourdough bread for a soothing, simple lunch. This recipe is also very good with almond butter or hazelnut butter instead of peanut butter. For a low-fat soup, omit the peanut butter.

1 three-pound butternut squash
2 cups vegetable broth
1/4 cup smooth peanut butter
1 teaspoon curry powder (or to taste)
2 cups unsweetened soy milk
salt to taste
optional garnishes: finely chopped peanuts, chopped scallions

Remove the peel and seeds from the squash and cut the flesh into large chunks. In a large saucepan, simmer squash in the vegetable broth, covered, until squash is tender (about fifteen to twenty minutes, depending on the size of the squash pieces). Allow squash to cool for a few minutes, then transfer squash and cooking broth to a blender container. Add peanut butter and curry powder and blend until very smooth. Add a little more liquid if necessary to facilitate blending. Return mixture to saucepan. Add soy milk, and heat through (do not boil). Salt to taste. Serve immediately. Makes 4 to 6 servings.

From Vegging Out

Soy Cassava Soup

2 cups cooked and mashed cassava
2 cups Okara or cooked and mashed soybeans
1 teaspoon salt
4–5 cups water
3 teaspoons soy oil
3 teaspoons chopped onion
1 teaspoon garlic paste
1/4 teaspoon black pepper

In a soup pan, fry oil, onion, garlic paste and pepper for two to three minutes. Add water, salt, soy, cassava and okara. Bring to boil, and adjust seasoning and thickness according to preference. Boil for five minutes on low heat. Serve warm. Variations: Potatoes, rice, corn and different vegetables can be used in soup preparation utilizing soybeans.

From INTSOY, University of Illinois at Urbana-Champaign

Salads

Creamy Herb Miso Dressing

1/2 cup low-fat soy milk
1/4 cup white miso
1/4 cup brown rice vinegar
1/4 cup onion, chopped
1 tablespoon fresh basil, chopped
1 tablespoon fresh tarragon, chopped

1 tablespoon fresh parsley, chopped
1 teaspoon honey
1 teaspoon Dijon mustard
1 teaspoon coriander powder

In a blender or food processor, blend all ingredients until smooth. Cover and refrigerate at least four hours to allow flavors to develop. Serve with your favorite salad greens. Makes 10 two-tablespoon servings.

From Ron Pickarski, CEC and the Indiana Soybean Board

Creamy Italian Dressing

1 cup plain soy milk
1 package (12 ounces) firm tofu
2 packages (0.7 ounce each) dry Italian dressing mix

Mix all ingredients in blender or food processor until smooth and creamy. Refrigerate. Makes 2 to 3 cups.

From the Indiana Soybean Board

Soy Caesar Salad with Parmesan Croutons

CROUTONS
2 slices bread
1 tablespoon soy or olive oil
2 tablespoons Parmesan cheese

Cut bread into small cubes. Toss bread with oil and Parmesan cheese until well blended. Place on ungreased baking sheet. Bake for ten minutes at 300°F until crisp. Set aside.

DRESSING
1/4 cup olive oil
3/4 cup soy milk

4 cloves garlic, minced
1/4 ounce anchovy paste
1/4 teaspoon kosher or sea salt
1/2 teaspoon cracked black pepper
1/2 teaspoon Worcestershire sauce
dash of lemon juice

Mix all ingredients together in mixing bowl until well blended. Refrigerate until well chilled. Blend again just before serving, if necessary.

SALAD
1 head Romaine lettuce, washed and dried on paper toweling

Tear washed lettuce into bite-size pieces. Place in salad bowl. Add croutons and dressing. Makes 6 servings.
From Chef Carrie Balkcom, CEC and Sous Chef Stacey E. Evans, CC

Cucumber, Tomato, Tofu Salad with Citrus Vinaigrette

SALAD
1 large cucumber, seeded, cut into thin slices
1/2 pound cherry tomatoes, rinsed, stemmed and cut in half
1/2 pound hard tofu, cut into small cubes

DRESSING
1/2 cup olive oil
1/4 cup rice wine vinegar
1/4 teaspoon sea or kosher salt
1/4 teaspoon cracked black pepper
1 teaspoon concentrated orange juice

Place prepared cucumber, tomatoes and tofu in medium bowl. Mix well. Combine dressing ingredients, and add to salad mixture. Mix well. Add soy sprouts. Mix gently. Serve immediately.
From Chef Carrie Balkcom, CEC and Sous Chef Stacey E. Evans, CC

Tasty Coleslaw

For extra bite, add a few drops of Tabasco sauce or a teaspoon of horseradish.

1/3 cup creamed tofu (mix with a little vinegar in blender)
2 tablespoons mayonnaise
2 tablespoons balsamic or rice vinegar
2 teaspoons brown sugar
1 teaspoon dry mustard
1 teaspoon celery seed
salt to taste
ground black pepper to taste
3 cups shredded green cabbage
1/3 cup shredded carrot
dash of red pepper

Mix creamed tofu, mayonnaise, vinegar, brown sugar, mustard, celery seed, salt and pepper in a large bowl. Add cabbage and carrots and toss until vegetables are evenly coated. Sprinkle with red pepper. Makes 4 servings.

From Rita Elkins

Crunchy Confetti Salad

For this salad, try to cut the vegetables all approximately the same size as the soybeans. Feel free to add or substitute other veggies, depending on what's available (try cucumber, radish, zucchini or celery).

1 tablespoon olive oil (optional)
1 tablespoon balsamic vinegar
1 1/2 cup cooked soybeans
2 bell peppers, trimmed and diced (for the prettiest effect, use two
    different colors, such as red and yellow, or orange and green)

1/2 red onion, diced
1/2 cup chopped fresh parsley
salt to taste (optional)

Whisk together olive oil and balsamic vinegar. Set aside. Combine soybeans, diced peppers and diced onion in a bowl. Add dressing and parsley, and toss to combine. Add salt to taste. Chill thoroughly before serving. Makes about 3 cups.

From Vegging Out

Seven-Layer Soybean Salad

A revision of an old potluck standby, this salad is beautiful and nutritious. Serve it in a glass bowl to show off the colors. The ingredient amounts will vary according to how many people you're serving and the size of your bowl—use whatever amounts look good!

boiled and sliced red salad potatoes
blanched broccoli florets (To blanch broccoli florets, boil them for
    one minute in water to cover, then drain immediately.)
shredded red cabbage
cooked soybeans
chopped Romaine lettuce
a thin layer of mayonnaise dressing
Lightlife Fakin' Bacon Bits or sunflower seeds

Arrange the ingredients in layers in the order listed above. Do not toss. Chill thoroughly before serving.

From Vegging Out

Vegetable Dishes

Mushrooms, Tofu and Snow Peas in Soy Ginger Sauce

1 small onion, halved and thinly sliced crosswise
1 tablespoon vegetable oil
1/4 pound mushrooms, thinly sliced
1 garlic clove, minced
2 teaspoons minced ginger root
3/4 teaspoon cornstarch dissolved in 2 tablespoons cold water
3 tablespoons soy sauce
1/2 pound firm tofu, drained, wrapped in a double thickness of
    paper towels for 15 minutes and cut into 1/4-inch thick slices
1/2 cup water
1/4 pound snow peas, no strings
cooked rice

Brown onions in a skillet over moderately high heat, stirring occasionally. Add the mushrooms and sauté the mixture, stirring until the mushrooms are tender. Add the garlic and the ginger and sauté the mixture, stirring for one minute. Stir the cornstarch mixture and add it to the skillet with the soy sauce, tofu and water. Simmer the mixture, stirring gently and turning tofu to coat with sauce. Add the snow peas and stir gently for thirty seconds. Serve over rice. Makes 2 servings.

From the Maryland Soybean Board

Soy and Veggie Napoleons

12 four-inch squares puff pastry, defrosted
1 eggplant, stemmed and cut into quarters
1 summer squash, stemmed and cut into slices
12 ounces soy cheese (mozzarella or your favorite)
1 bunch green onion, chopped coarsely

3 or 4 Roma tomatoes cut into 12 round slices
6 to 8 fresh basil leaves, washed and torn in half

Place eggplant and squash on baking sheet and brush with olive oil. Cook at 350°F for twenty minutes. Let cool. Take one square of puff pastry and place on pastry in the following order eggplant, squash mixture, green onion, soy cheese, tomato and basil. Fold pastry over to form a triangle. Pinch edges together. With wet fingers, seal the edges on the puff pastry.

Heat oven to 375°F. Place completed Napoleons on an ungreased baking sheet and bake twenty-five minutes until golden brown. Makes 12 servings.

From Chef Carrie Balkcom, CEC and Sous Chef Stacey E. Evans, CC;
adapted from The Whole Soy Cook Book

Soy Spanokopita

1 pound cooked frozen spinach, thawed and drained
1 tablespoon soybean oil
3 tablespoons butter
1 small onion, finely chopped
1 tablespoon chopped garlic
10 ounces soy cheese (any variety)
1 tablespoon lemon pepper
sea or kosher salt and cracked black pepper to taste
5 sheets filo pastry
2 ounces melted butter

Thaw and drain spinach in colander. Set aside. Preheat oven to 350°F. Heat oil and butter in saucepan and add onion and garlic. Cook gently for two minutes. Remove from heat and add half of the drained spinach. Add half of the soy cheese. Mix well. Add spices and seasonings to taste. Mix in remaining spinach and cheese. Lay one sheet of pastry on work surface. Brush with butter. Cover with second sheet, continuing until all five sheets are used. Spread filling over pastry, leaving a one-inch border. Roll in sides jelly-roll style. Place roll seam side-down on a greased baking sheet and brush with butter. Bake in 350°F oven for thirty minutes until golden brown. Makes 4 servings.

From Chef Carrie Balkcom, CEC and Sous Chef Stacey E. Evans, CC

Potato Rags

12 ounces shredded hash brown potatoes
soybean oil, as needed
2 ounces diced onion
2 ounces shredded cheddar cheese
2 ounces shredded mozzarella or provolone cheese
3 ounces prepared ranch-style dressing
3 ounces diced tomatoes
2 ounces cooked bacon, crumbled

Deep-fry the hash browns in soybean oil at 375°F until lightly browned. Drain well. Place fried hash brown on serving platter. Top with onion and cheeses. Microwave at high for about thirty seconds, or until cheese melts. Top with ranch dressing, tomatoes and bacon. Makes 2 to 4 servings.

From Mark D. Rogers, president, Habits Café, Cincinnati

Roasted Garlic Soybean Hummus

Made with soybeans instead of the traditional garbanzo beans, this hummus is rich with the taste of roasted garlic. Make it thick to spread on bread or crackers or thin to use as a dip.

3 large cloves of garlic
1 1/2 cups cooked soybeans
2 tablespoons roasted sesame tahini
1 tablespoon olive oil
1 tablespoon lemon juice
1/2 cup fresh parsley

1 to 4 tablespoons water or vegetable broth
salt to taste

Preheat broiler. Broil garlic cloves for five to ten minutes or until they just begin to brown and can be pierced easily with a fork. In a food processor, combine garlic with soybeans, tahini, olive oil, lemon juice and parsley. Blend until smooth, adding salt to taste and water or broth to reach desired consistency. Makes about one and one half cups.

From Vegging Out

Winter Squash Soufflé

2 pounds cooked, mashed, drained squash (any variety)
1/3 cup melted butter
1/4 cup sugar
1/3 cup soy milk
2 eggs, beaten
1/4 teaspoon dried dill
1/4 teaspoon nutmeg

Peel and quarter squash and boil until tender. Drain and mash with fork. In a 2-quart baking dish, pour melted butter. Coat sides and let the rest of the butter settle to the bottom. Add sugar, soy milk, eggs, spices and squash. Mix well. Bake at 350° F for thirty to forty-five minutes until center is set. Makes 6 servings.

From Chef Carrie Balkcom, CEC and Sous Chef Stacey E. Evans, CC

Soybean and Eggplant Summer Gratin

This recipe began with an idea for vegetarian moussaka and evolved into a simple and colorful summer casserole that's good warm or at room temperature. You can substitute garbanzo beans for the soybeans.

1 tablespoon olive oil
1 onion, chopped
3 cloves garlic, minced
3 four-inch baby eggplants or 1 medium eggplant, trimmed and
    diced in 1/2-inch pieces
1/2 teaspoon paprika
1/4 teaspoon nutmeg
1/4 teaspoon salt
6 plums or Roma tomatoes, chopped
1 1/2 cups cooked soybeans
1 1/2 cups fresh bread crumbs

Preheat oven to 350° F. Sauté onion and garlic in olive oil for one minute. Add eggplant, and sauté for five to ten minutes, or until eggplant is soft. Stir in paprika, nutmeg and salt. Transfer contents of sauté pan to a 2 1/2-quart casserole dish. Add chopped tomatoes and soybeans, and stir to combine. Sprinkle bread crumbs over the top. Bake casserole, covered, for thirty minutes. Uncover, and bake fifteen more minutes, or until top is lightly browned. Makes 4–6 servings.

From Vegging Out

Soy Style Refried Beans (Tutu)

5 cups soft cooked soybeans
1/2 cup chopped onion
1/2 cup chopped tomatoes
1 teaspoon garlic paste
2–3 cups water
1 teaspoon salt
1 chopped green bell pepper (optional)
1/2 teaspoon black pepper
cassava flour (approximately 1 cup)
1/3 cup green onion, chopped
3 tablespoons chopped parsley
2 hard-cooked eggs, sliced (optional)

stir-fry collard leaves (optional)
1/3 cup soy oil

Heat oil. Add onions, tomatoes, black pepper, green pepper, garlic paste and salt. Add soybeans, and mash as much as possible. Add water and let boil. Add cassava flour (a little at a time), stirring frequently. Adjust seasoning to taste. Put mixture in a serving dish. Decorate with collard leaves, parsley or boiled eggs.

From INTSOY, University of Illinois at Urbana-Champaign

Main Dishes

Soy-Style Lasagna

1 pound ground beef
1/2 cup chopped onions
1 jar spaghetti sauce
1 container (16 ounces) ricotta cheese
1 eight-ounce package firm tofu
3 cups shredded mozzarella cheese, divided
1/2 cup Parmesan cheese, plus extra
2 eggs
1 tablespoon chopped fresh parsley
1/2 teaspoon salt
1/4 teaspoon garlic powder
1/4 teaspoon pepper
1 box lasagna noodles

Brown meat and onions, and drain. Add sauce. Combine ricotta cheese, tofu, 1 1/2 cups mozzarella cheese, Parmesan cheese, eggs, parsley, salt, garlic powder and pepper for the filling. Spread enough tomato sauce into bottom of 9 inch x 13 inch pan to keep noodles from sticking; place dry uncooked lasagna noodles in a single layer across bottom of pan. Top with a layer of cheese mixture; spread sauce over cheese mixture, and alternate layers with noodles. Layer to near top of pan. Pour about one cup of water carefully along the side of the dish.

Cover with aluminum foil and bake at 350°F for thirty to forty-five minutes or until hot and bubbly and noodles are soft. Uncover; spread remaining mozzarella cheese over lasagna and sprinkle with Parmesan cheese. Bake about ten minutes longer or until mozzarella topping is melted or lightly browned. Let stand about ten minutes before cutting for easier serving.

From the Soy Connection

Pasta with Sweet Beans, Bell Peppers and Basil

1 tablespoon soy oil
1 cup chopped onion
1/2 teaspoon fennel seeds, crushed
2 cloves garlic, minced
2 cups frozen green soybeans
2 fourteen and one half-ounce cans diced tomatoes, no salt added, undrained
1 pound yellow bell peppers, roasted and peeled
1/2 teaspoon salt
1/4 teaspoon freshly ground pepper
1 pound penne rigatoni (short tubular pasta)
1/2 cup fresh basil, chopped
1/2 cup grated Parmesan cheese

Heat oil in a large nonstick skillet over medium-low heat. Add onion, fennel seeds and garlic; cover and cook five minutes, stirring occasionally. Add tomatoes and bring to a boil. Reduce heat and simmer uncovered for twenty minutes.

Cut peppers in half, and clean out the seeds. Arrange peppers in a single layer on a baking sheet. Place in the oven under the broiler. Broil peppers until they are blistered and charred on all sides, about ten minutes. Remove and place in a heavy paper bag, close the end and let them sweat for five to ten minutes. Scrape off charred skins. Cut into julienne strips about two inches long.

Bring a large pot of water to boil for the pasta. Add pasta and cook according to package directions, about nine to ten minutes. Add bell pepper strips, green soybeans, salt and pepper to tomato mixture; cover and cook for five minutes. Serve pasta topped with the tomato mixture and basil. Sprinkle with grated Parmesan cheese.

From the Maryland Soybean Board

Herb-Crusted Roasted Pork Loin Stuffed with Soy Sausage

1 tablespoon dried oregano
1 tablespoon dried thyme
1 tablespoon garlic powder
1 tablespoon crushed black pepper
1 tablespoon sea or kosher salt
1 to 1 1/2 pounds pork loin
1 pound soy sausage

Freeze soy sausage. Mix dried spices and set aside. With a boning knife, cut a hole in the middle of the pork loin (or have the butcher do it for you).

Push the frozen soy sausage into the hole, and push until all sausage is in the cavity. Put dried spice mixture into a baking pan. Roll the stuffed pork loin in the dried spice mixture. Wrap the pork in aluminum foil tightly. Bake in preheated 350°F oven for forty-five minutes to one hour until done or until internal temperature reads 160°F. Remove from oven and let sit. Cut into medium slices and serve.

From Chef Carrie Balkcom, CEC and Sous Chef Stacey E. Evans, CC

Chili Fest

1 package soy burgers
1 package chili seasoning mix
1 medium onion, chopped
1 green pepper, coarsely chopped
3 cloves minced garlic
1 sixteen-ounce can crushed tomatoes
1 sixteen-ounce can tomato sauce
1 sixteen-ounce can pinto beans
1 sixteen-ounce can red beans
2 tablespoons chili powder
3/4 teaspoon cumin
1/4 teaspoon cayenne pepper
salt and pepper to tasted

Cook the burgers. Combine the rest of the ingredients in a large pot. Crumble the cooked patties and add to chili mixture. Simmer for thirty minutes.

From Rita Elkins

Tri-Colored Fusilli Pasta with Soy Cream Sauce and Wild Mushroom Ragout

1 pound tri-color fusilli pasta

WILD MUSHROOM RAGOUT AND SAUCE
1 pound assorted wild mushrooms, cut into medium pieces
2 tablespoons minced garlic
1/2 small onion, diced
2 cups soy milk
3 ounces butter
1/4 cup flour
salt and pepper to taste
1/4 cup chopped fresh parsley
Parmesan cheese to taste

Cook pasta according to package directions and set aside. In medium shallow pan, melt butter slowly over low heat. Add flour until well mixed. Add soy milk, and reduce heat by one third. Add wild mushrooms, onion and garlic. Stir in well, but do not overwork. Cover and let steam five to ten minutes over low heat. Season with salt and pepper. Add cooked pasta to mushroom mixture and mix well. Pour into serving bowl and garnish with chopped parsley and Parmesan cheese. Makes 6 servings.

From Chef Carrie Balkcom, CEC and Sous Chef Stacey E. Evans, CC

Textured Soy Protein Tacos

1 cup dry textured soy protein (TSP)
7/8 cup boiling water
1 1/2 cups tomato sauce
1 1/2 teaspoons chili powder
1 1/2 teaspoons garlic
1 teaspoon sugar
8 corn tortillas
chopped tomatoes, lettuce and salsa

Pour the boiling water over the TSP and set aside. Combine the tomato sauce, chili powder, garlic and sugar, and simmer for ten minutes. Add the TSP and cook for another ten minutes. Serve in warmed tortilla shells topped with lettuce, tomatoes and salsa. Makes 8 tacos.

From Simply Soy

Broccoli Cheddar Cheese Wedges

16 ounces frozen chopped broccoli, thawed
1/2 cup chopped onion
2 cups (8 ounces) cheddar soy cheese, shredded
1 1/4 cups plain soy milk
3 egg whites

1 tablespoon vegetable oil
3/4 cup soy flour
1 teaspoon baking powder
1 tablespoon dried parsley
1 tablespoon minced garlic
1/4 teaspoon pepper

Preheat oven to 400°F. Lightly coat a ten or eleven-inch pie dish or casserole dish with vegetable cooking spray. Layer the broccoli, onion and cheddar soy cheese in dish. Combine all remaining ingredients in blender and mix until smooth. Pour over vegetable/cheese mixture and bake for about thirty to forty minutes, until lightly browned and knife inserted near center comes out clean. Cool five minutes before cutting into wedges. Makes 8 wedges.

From the Indiana Soybean Board

Grilled Polenta with Tomato Coulis

POLENTA
2 quarts soy milk
1 teaspoon salt
1 1/2 cups polenta
2 tablespoons butter
1/4 cup Parmesan cheese

COULIS
1 fourteen-ounce can crushed tomatoes
1 chopped onion
1 teaspoon butter
1 tablespoon crushed garlic
1/8 teaspoon dried sage

In a large saucepan, bring soy milk to gentle boil. Stir in salt. While stirring, add polenta slowly until mixture has thickened. Lower heat and simmer ten minutes, stirring frequently. Add butter, Parmesan cheese and coulis seasonings. Pour mixture into a lightly greased, shallow baking dish. Chill until set. Makes 6 servings.

From Chef Carrie Balkcom, CEC and Sous Chef Stacey E. Evans, CC

Chunky Barbecue Tempeh

Serve this versatile dish over noodles or rice or with thick slices of French bread. For a low-fat version, sauté the onions and garlic in water or vegetable broth instead of oil.

2 tablespoons olive oil
1 medium onion, coarsely chopped
3 cloves garlic, minced
1 14-ounce can unsalted tomatoes, drained and coarsely chopped
2 tablespoons honey, molasses, or maple syrup
2 tablespoons brown rice vinegar or cider vinegar
2 tablespoons tamari
1 teaspoon paprika
1 teaspoon ground cumin
8 ounces tempeh, steamed for twenty minutes and cut in
  1-inch strips, 1/4-inch thick

In a medium saucepan, sauté onion and garlic in olive oil for five minutes. Add remaining ingredients and simmer, partially covered, for fifteen to twenty minutes, or until sauce thickens. Makes 4 servings.

From Vegging Out

Breads

Pumpkin Bread

2/3 cup sifted soy flour
3/4 teaspoon salt
1 cup sifted all-purpose flour
1/4 cup soy oil
1/4 teaspoon baking powder
1 1/4 cups sugar
3/4 teaspoon baking soda
4 egg whites, well beaten
1 1/2 teaspoons cinnamon
3/4 cup canned pumpkin
1/2 teaspoon ground cloves
2 tablespoons water
1/4 teaspoon nutmeg

Sift and measure soy flour and all-purpose flour. Measure other dry ingredients except sugar, and sift together with flour. Set aside. Cream soy oil and sugar together. Add egg whites and beat until light. Blend in pumpkin and water. Add dry ingredients in two portions, blending well. Pour batter into greased 9 inch x 5 inch x 3 inch inch loaf pan. Bake at 350°F for sixty-five to seventy minutes. Remove loaf from pan immediately and cool on a wire rack.

From the United Soybean Board

Oatmeal Bread (Bread Machine)

3 cups bread flour
1/3 cup soy flour
3 tablespoons sugar
1 1/2 teaspoons salt
1 1/2 tablespoons margarine
1/3 cup oatmeal

3/4 cup soy milk (plain or vanilla)
3/4 cup water
1 1/2 teaspoons dry yeast

Add ingredients to bread machine according to manufacturer's directions. All ingredients should be at room temperature for best results. Makes 1 loaf (about 1 1/2 pounds).

From the Indiana Soybean Board

Zesty Cornbread Muffins

3/4 cup all purpose flour
1/4 cup soy flour
1 cup yellow cornmeal
1/4 cup sugar
4 teaspoons baking powder
1 teaspoon salt
1 teaspoon chili powder
1 cup plain soy milk
1/4 cup vegetable oil
2 eggs, slightly beaten
3/4 cup shredded reduced fat cheddar cheese
1/4 cup chopped green chilies
1/4 cup chopped jalapeño peppers

Preheat oven to 425°F. Coat muffin pan with vegetable cooking spray. In medium bowl, combine flours, cornmeal, sugar, baking powder, salt and chili powder. In a separate bowl, stir together soy milk, oil and eggs. Add to dry ingredients and blend slightly. Stir in cheese, chilies and peppers. Pour into muffin pan. Bake for eighteen to twenty-four minutes or until toothpick inserted in center comes out clean. Remove muffins from pan and cool on wire rack.

CORNBREAD VERSION: Place batter in greased 8-inch round or square baking pan. Cook eighteen to twenty-two minutes. Cool on wire rack. Cut into twelve pieces. Makes 12 muffins.

From the Indiana Soybean Board

Blueberry Muffins

1 1/2 cups flour (may be all or part whole wheat)
1/2 cup soy flour
2 teaspoons baking powder
1/3 cup brown sugar
1/2 teaspoon cinnamon
1 cup soy milk
2 egg whites
2 tablespoons soybean oil
1 cup blueberries

Preheat oven to 375° F. In a large mixing bowl, stir together well the flour, soy flour, baking powder, brown sugar and cinnamon. In a small mixing bowl, whisk together the soy milk, egg whites and oil. Pour into the dry ingredients and mix just until blended. Stir the blueberries into the batter (if using frozen berries, do not thaw first). Divide batter among twelve nonstick or lightly greased muffin cups. Bake at 375°F for fifteen to eighteen minutes, until golden and the center tests done. Remove from pan immediately. Makes 12 muffins.

From the Indiana Soybean Board

Lemon Poppy Seed Muffins

1 3/4 cups all-purpose flour
1/2 cup soy flour
1 teaspoon baking powder
1 teaspoon baking soda
1/8 teaspoon salt
1 package (12 ounces) soft silken tofu
3/4 cup sugar
1/4 cup vegetable oil
1 egg
2 egg whites
1 tablespoon lemon juice

3 tablespoons vanilla soy milk
3 tablespoons poppy seeds
1 tablespoon lemon zest

Preheat oven to 375°F. In a large mixing bowl, mix together flours, baking soda and powder, and salt. In a smaller bowl, whisk together tofu and sugar until crumbled. Add oil, egg, egg whites, lemon juice, soy milk, poppy seeds and lemon zest and mix with a fork or spoon until well blended. Add this liquid mixture to dry ingredients and mix only until all ingredients are moistened and combined. Spray muffin cups with vegetable cooking spray and place batter in cups; fill each about two-thirds full. Bake fifteen to twenty-five minutes or until done. Makes 12 muffins.

From the Indiana Soybean Board

Desserts

Cherry Tofu Delight

1 eight-ounce package low-fat cream cheese, softened
1 package (10.5 ounces) firm tofu
1 eight-ounce container lite Cool Whip
1 can cherry pie filling

Blend cream cheese and tofu in blender until smooth. Fold in Cool Whip. Mix in pie filling and spoon into parfait glasses. Refrigerate until set. Serve with garnish. (Cholesterol content may be reduced by substituting cream cheese with all tofu.) Makes 16 servings.

From the Maryland Soybean Board

Peach Cobbler Cake

3/4 cup flour (all or part whole-wheat)
1/4 cup soy flour
2 teaspoons baking powder
1/2 teaspoon cinnamon
1/2 teaspoon nutmeg
1/2 cup sugar
2/3 cup soy milk
1/4 teaspoon almond extract
1 can (16 ounce) sliced peaches, drained well and cut
    into half-inch pieces

Preheat the oven to 350°F. In a medium bowl, combine the flour, soy flour, baking powder, cinnamon, nutmeg and sugar. Stir together well. Add soy milk and almond extract and stir just until blended. Gently stir in the drained and chopped peaches. Pour the batter into an 8-inch square baking pan coated with nonstick spray. Bake at 350°F for thirty-five to forty minutes, until a toothpick inserted in the center comes out clean. Cut into squares. Makes 9 servings.

From Simply Soy

Gingerbread

This moist gingerbread is made extra special with fresh ginger, but you can substitute dried ginger if you prefer. Great for the holidays!

1/3 cup brown sugar
1/2 cup molasses
1/2 cup warm soy milk
1/4 cup applesauce
6 tablespoons grated fresh ginger or 2 teaspoons dried ginger
2 egg whites
2/3 cup all-purpose flour

1/2 cup whole-wheat flour
1/3 cup soy flour
1/2 teaspoon cinnamon
1/2 teaspoon allspice
1 teaspoon baking soda

Preheat the oven to 350°F. Using an electric mixer, combine the brown sugar, molasses and warm soy milk in a bowl. Beat in the applesauce, fresh ginger (if using) and egg whites. Sift together the three flours, cinnamon, allspice and baking soda (and dried ginger, if using). Add to the liquid ingredients and beat just until smooth. Pour into a nonstick or lightly greased eight-inch square pan and bake at 350°F for about thirty minutes, until the center tests done and edges pull away from the sides of the pan. Cut into nine squares and serve warm or at room temperature. Makes 9 servings.

From Simply Soy

Soy Brownies

1/2 cup sifted all-purpose flour
1/4 cup sifted soy flour
1/2 teaspoon salt
1/2 teaspoon baking powder
1/3 cup vegetable shortening
1 cup sugar
2 eggs*
1/2 teaspoon vanilla
2 squares unsweetened chocolate, melted*
1/2 cup chopped soy nuts

Sift together twice the all-purpose flour, soy flour, baking powder and salt. Cream shortening; gradually blend in sugar and all well-beaten eggs. Beat until smooth and fluffy. Add vanilla and stir in melted chocolate. Add flour mixture in three portions, stirring after each addition. Add nuts. Pour into an 8-inch square greased pan. Bake at 325°F for twenty-five to thirty minutes. Cut into squares and serve.

*By replacing two egg whites for each whole egg and using three tablespoons Dutch processed cocoa powder per one square unsweetened chocolate, you can reduce fat to 4.14 grams; cholesterol to 0 milligrams; and calories to 100.) Makes about 20 brownies.

From the Maryland Soybean Board

Chocolate Chip Oatmeal Cookies

3 egg whites, lightly beaten
1/2 cup brown sugar
1/2 cup granulated sugar
2 teaspoons vanilla
1/3 cup soynut butter
2 medium bananas, mashed (about 1 cup)
1 1/2 cups flour (may be all or part whole-wheat)
1/2 cup soy flour
1 1/2 teaspoons baking powder
1/2 cups soy milk
1 1/2 cups dry oats
1 package (6 ounces) chocolate chips

Preheat the oven to 375°F In a large mixing bowl, beat together egg whites, brown sugar, granulated sugar, vanilla, soynut butter and bananas. Sift together flour, soy flour and baking powder. Stir about half the dry mixture into the banana mixture, stir in the soy milk, and then mix in the rest of the flour mixture. Stir in the oats and chocolate chips. Drop the dough by teaspoonfuls about one and one half-inch apart on nonstick or lightly greased cookie sheets. Bake at 375°F for ten to twelve minutes or until lightly browned around the edges. Remove cookies to wire rack to cool. Makes about 5 dozen cookies.

From Simply Soy

Best Ever Snickerdoodles

1/2 cup margarine, softened
1/2 cup soy flour, sifted
1/2 cup all-purpose flour
1 cup sugar
1 egg
1/2 teaspoon vanilla
1/4 teaspoon baking soda
1/2 teaspoon baking powder
1/2 cup wheat flour, whole-grain
2 tablespoons sugar
1 teaspoon cinnamon

Mix margarine on high speed for thirty seconds. Add soy flour, all-purpose flour, one cup sugar, egg, vanilla, baking soda and baking powder. Beat together. Beat in the whole-wheat flour.

Chill dough for one hour. Shape into one-inch balls. Roll the balls in sugar/cinnamon mixture and place on a greased cookie sheet. Bake at 375°F for ten minutes. Cool on a wire rack. Makes approximately 40 cookies.

From Kristen Dougherty/the Indiana Soybean Board

Caramel Surprise Pudding

Kids love the surprises in this pudding! The pudding will be even sweeter if you make it with vanilla soy milk.

4 graham cracker squares
1/2 medium banana
2 tablespoons brown sugar
3 tablespoons cornstarch
1 1/2 cups plain or vanilla soy milk
1/4 cup fat-free caramel topping
1 teaspoon vanilla

Break each graham cracker square into four pieces and cut banana into small chunks. Put the grapham cracker pieces and banana chunks in a medium serving bowl or divide among four small serving dishes.

Combine the brown sugar and cornstarch in a medium saucepan. Stir in the soy milk and caramel topping. Cook, stirring, over moderate heat until pudding just comes to a boil and thickens. Remove from heat and stir in vanilla. Pour the pudding over the graham crackers and bananas and stir well. Cover and refrigerate. Serve the pudding well chilled. Makes 4 half-cup servings.

From Simply Soy

Raspberry Sherbet

3/4 cup soy milk
3/4 cup cranberry-raspberry juice
1 cup raspberries, puréed
2 tablespoons sugar

Blend all ingredients and freeze in an ice cream maker or in the freezer (directions below).

Ice cream maker: Freeze according to manufacturer's recommendations. This recipe fits a one-pint ice cream maker. You can double the recipe for larger machines.

Freezer: Pour into a shallow pan and freeze until fairly firm but not totally frozen. Cut into chunks and process in a food processor or blender until smooth. Pour into a container and freeze again. Let soften before serving. If necessary, process again briefly just before serving. Makes 2 cups (4 servings).

From Simply Soy

Spice Drop Cookies

1 cup brown sugar
1/4 cup soy oil

1 jar (2.5 ounces) prune baby food or 1/4 cup prune purée
2 egg whites
1/2 cup applesauce
1 teaspoon vanilla
1 cup cooked soybeans, rinsed, drained and mashed
2 cups flour (may use all or part whole-wheat)
2 teaspoons baking powder
1 teaspoon cinnamon
1/2 teaspoon nutmeg
1/4 teaspoon cloves
1/4 teaspoon ginger
1 cup oats
1 cup raisins

Preheat the oven to 375°F. Combine the brown sugar, oil, prune baby food, egg whites, applesauce and vanilla in a large mixing bowl. Beat together well with an electric mixer. Beat in the mashed soybeans. In a medium mixing bowl, sift together the flour, baking powder, cinnamon, nutmeg, cloves and ginger. Stir them into the soybean mixture. Stir the oats and raisins into the dough.

Drop the dough by rounded teaspoonfuls onto a nonstick (or lightly greased) baking sheet. Bake at 375°F for ten minutes, until firm and lightly golden.

PUMPKIN SPICE COOKIES: Substitute mashed cooked pumpkin for the applesauce. Makes about 5 dozen (60) cookies.

From Simply Soy

Instant Chocolate Mousse

1 box instant chocolate pudding mix (four-serving size)
1 1/4 cups cold soy milk
1 package (10.5 ounces) silken tofu

Put the contents of the chocolate pudding mix and the soy milk into a blender and whirl until very smooth, about fifteen seconds. Add the silken tofu and blend again, scraping down sides as needed, until very smooth. Pour into individual serving dishes and chill at least two hours before serving. Makes 4 half-cup servings.

From Simply Soy

Decadent Dip

Nutella® is a chocolate hazelnut spread that is available in gourmet stores and many supermarkets.

1 package (10.5 ounces) silken tofu
6 tablespoons Nutella®

Whirl the silken tofu and Nutella® together in a blender, scraping down sides as needed. Put into a serving dish and serve with fresh fruit or dipping size chunks of banana bread. Makes 5 half-cup servings.

From Simply Soy

Silken Tofu Cheesecake

1/4 cup graham cracker crumbs (four squares)
1 package (10.5 ounces) silken tofu
3/4 cup liquid egg substitute
1/2 cup sugar
1 tablespoon lemon juice
1 teaspoon vanilla extract
1 cup nonfat ricotta cheese

Preheat the oven to 325°F. Spray an eight-inch springform pan or eight-inch pie pan with vegetable oil spray. Evenly spread graham cracker crumbs on the bottom of the pan. Drain the tofu well. Put it into a blender along with the egg substitute, sugar, lemon juice, vanilla and nonfat ricotta cheese. Blend until smooth, scraping down sides as necessary. Pour the tofu mixture into the prepared pan and bake at 325°F for thirty-five to forty minutes. Remove from the oven and cool fifteen minutes at room temperature. Refrigerate. Decorate with your favorite fresh fruits, if desired. Cut into wedges to serve. Makes 8 servings.

From Simply Soy

Tiramisu

Savoiardi biscuits, or Italian ladyfinger cookies, are sold in Italian food stores. Other ladyfinger cookies will work, as well. The tofu amounts used are not hard and fast either, so if your package weighs a few ounces more or less, go ahead and use it.

16 ounces silken tofu
1/2 cup tofu cream cheese
1/3 cup sugar
2 tablespoons dark rum
1 to 2 tablespoons brandy
2 teaspoons lemon juice
1 cup cold espresso coffee
20 Savoiardi biscuits or other brand of ladyfinger cookies
1 ounce dark chocolate, grated
1/2 ounce dark chocolate, chopped

In a food processor, puree tofu until smooth. Line a strainer with paper towels and place over a bowl. Pour tofu into strainer and refrigerate while it drains for two to three hours. (One fourth-cup of liquid should collect in the bowl.) Pour drained tofu back into food processor. Add cream cheese, sugar, half of the rum, the brandy and lemon juice, and process to blend well. In a large bowl, combine coffee and remaining rum. Quickly dip biscuits into coffee mixture, one by one. Turn to coat, and place each into an eight-inch square baking dish, covering bottom in a single layer, about ten cookies. (Working quickly will keep the biscuits from soaking up too much liquid.)

Spread half of the tofu mixture over cookies. Sprinkle half of the grated chocolate over top. Repeat layers with remaining ingredients. Sprinkle chopped chocolate over top, cover and refrigerate for at least two hours (up to twenty-four hours). Makes 9 servings.

From the United Soy Board

Tofu Pumpkin Pie

This is great for a holiday dinner! You can also serve this as a crustless pumpkin pudding.

1 package (10.5 ounces) firm silken tofu
1 can (15 ounces) mashed pumpkin
1/2 cup brown sugar
1/4 cup white sugar
1 teaspoon ground cinnamon
1/2 teaspoon ground ginger
1/4 teaspoon ground cloves
1/4 teaspoon ground nutmeg
1 unbaked 9-inch pie shell (see Soy Oil Pie Crust)

Preheat oven to 425°. Drain tofu well, then purée in a blender until smooth. In a mixing bowl, whisk together the pumpkin and the sugars. Whisk in the spices and the puréed tofu. Pour the mixture into the pie shell and bake at 425°F for fifteen minutes. Lower the heat to 350°F and bake for an additional forty minutes. Chill before cutting into eighths and serving. Makes 1 nine-inch pie (eight wedges).

From Simply Soy

Cran-Apple Crumb

For this recipe, use old-fashioned rolled oats; the quick cooking or instant kinds won't produce a crisp topping. Tart Granny Smith apples provide the perfect contrast to the berries and nuts.

1/2 cup dried cranberries
1/3 cup raisins
1/2 cup orange juice
2 pounds Granny Smith apples, peeled, cored and cut into half-inch slices
1/2 cup raw or granulated sugar
1 teaspoon grated orange zest
1/2 teaspoon ground cinnamon
1 cup lite vanilla soy milk
1/2 cup rolled oats
1/2 cup unbleached white flour
1/2 cup dark brown sugar
1/4 teaspoon ground nutmeg
3 tablespoons cold unsalted butter or margarine
1/4 cup chopped walnuts
cooking spray

Preheat oven to 350°F. Lightly spray a deep, eight-cup baking dish with cooking spray. In a small bowl, soak cranberries and raisins in orange juice for twenty minutes; drain well. In a large bowl, combine apples, sugar, orange zest, cinnamon and drained fruit and toss to coat fruit well. Transfer to prepared baking dish and pour soy milk over apple mixture. In another large bowl, stir together oats, flour, brown sugar and nutmeg. Cut in butter or margarine, to a coarse, crumbly texture. Stir in walnuts. Sprinkle topping over apple mixture and pat lightly to form a rough crust. Bake until topping turns golden and apples are tender when a knife is inserted, about fifty to sixty minutes. Cool fifteen to twenty minute before serving. Makes 10 servings.

From the United Soy Board

Soy Oil Pie Crust

This crust is much lower in saturated fat than crusts made with butter or solid fats.

1 cup all-purpose flour (may use up to 1/2 cup whole-wheat flour)
1/4 cup soy oil
2 tablespoons plus 1 teaspoon cold water

Put the flour into a small mixing bowl. Add the soy oil and water and immediately stir with a fork. Make sure that all the flour is incorporated, and form dough into a ball. Flatten ball and place between two sheets of waxed paper. Roll out to a circle one inch bigger on all sides than the inverted pie pan (use 8-inch or 9-inch pie pan). Remove top sheet of waxed paper and invert pastry into pie pan. Remove remaining sheet of paper, smooth the pastry to fit the pan, and crimp the edges. Fill with pie filling and bake, or bake at 425°F for about fifteen minutes. Makes 1 eight-inch or nine-inch pie shell. Recipe may be doubled for a two-crust pie.

From Simply Soy

Appendix

Doctor to Doctor

Although much of this information has already been discussed, the following letter (from Dr. Neil Solomon) is specifically addressed to physicians and other health professionals and deals with current controversial clinical data on soy and its implications.

Dear Doctor or Health Professional,

During the thirty plus years that I practiced endocrinology, I treated over 30,000 patients with hormonally driven problems, many of whom suffered from estrogen-related maladies. During this time, I never really appreciated the effects of soy on women's health. Things have changed. While I have complete confidence in the health benefits of the soy bean for human health, conflicting data raises some controversy surrounding the use of soy. For this reason, I was particularly pleased to read Dr. Richard Hoeckh's balanced article on the subject of soy, which appeared in the February 2000 issue of *Integrative Medicine's, Herb & Dietary Supplement Report.* Using the work of Dr. Davis and his colleagues, he defines phytoestrogens as plant-derived compounds of nonsteroidal structure that possess estrogen-like biological activity.

According to Dr. Davis, there are three main classes of phytoestrogens: lignans, coumestans, and isoflavones. In this book, we chiefly address the soy isoflavone genistein, which is found along with daidzein primarily in legumes, and particularly in soybeans. As we discussed, it has been estimated that people in the Western culture consume less than five milligrams of isoflavones daily, while Asians consume 20 to 150 milligrams per day. It is well documented that the incidence of cardiovascular disease, breast and prostate cancer are lower in Asia than in Western countries.

I recently returned from a lecture tour in Southeast Asia, where it was suggested from both sides of the ocean that dietary factors play an important role in these statistical differences. This is in keeping with the published work of Dr. Davis. Is there any scientific evidence to suggest that isolated soy protein (ISP) inhibits cancer cell growth, increases bone density, and decreases hot flashes? The answer based on data points to "yes," because current scientific evidence seems to be heavily weighted on the positive side.

Dr. Davis and his associates conducted cell line studies done outside the body that suggest genistein may inhibit cancer cell growth by interfering with certain enzymes like tyrosine kinase. It appears that genistein exhibits a two-phase response (biphasic), resulting in a positive response (agonism) with estrogen receptors (ER) at low concentrations, and a negative ER response (antagonism) at increased concentrations.

The scientific team reports that the significance of the biphasic effect of genistein has not yet been established. Naturally, it would be helpful to know if other isoflavones also exhibit a biphasic effect. The Davis study looked at population studies (epidemiological) and found that women in Japan had a lower incidence, fewer nodal metastasis, and better prognosis with breast cancer than women in the United States.

In 1998, Dr. McMichael-Phillips and his colleagues, however, found inconsistencies in the epidemiological data showing a relationship between the high intake of soy in Japan and the low incidence of breast cancer. Their results are at odds with most of the other epidemiological published data. Dr. McMichael-Phillips conducted a randomly designed trial on forty-eight premenopausal women with benign breast disease or breast cancer, where half of the women consumed their normal diet, and the other half consumed their normal diet with the addition of 60 grams per day of textured soy protein containing 45 milligrams of isoflavones, for 14 days. In the soy group there was an increased growth rate of lobular epithelium breast tissue and progesterone receptor expression.

This raises questions about short-term (14 days), high-dose (60 grams per day of textured soy protein containing 45 milligrams of isoflavones) soy protein diet in premenopausal women with breast disease. The data is consistent with the possibility that soy may have different and opposite effects in premenopausal and postmenopausal women. The same may be true in ER positive or negative breast cancer patients, and those on tamoxifen.

So where does that leave us? It is important to realize that there are numerous factors affecting the outcome of adding soy to your diet. The safety of adding soy to the diet has not been established for postmenopausal women with ER positive breast cancer, women on tamoxifen, or premenopausal women with breast disease. On the other hand, no one has demonstrated that it is harmful for these people to add soy to their diet, and some believe that it is most likely beneficial. This seems to be an area that calls for more investigation. To date, the Asian model with its positive epidemiological data is our best model.

The effect of ISP on spinal bone density was studied by Dr. Potter and his team in 1998 on sixty-six postmenopausal women during a six-month, controlled, double-blind study. There were three parallel groups which given the following each day. (Group One: 40 grams of non-soy-based protein. Group Two: 40 grams ISP with 55.6 milligrams isoflavones. Group Three: 40 grams ISP with 90 milligrams isoflavones.) Group Three, with the addition of 90 milligrams/day showed a statistically significant increase in bone density. This data is solid when it comes to increasing bone density, but at present, there is still no documented evidence that increased soy intake is associated with a reduction in spinal fracture risk. Moreover, we still lack evidence to show that isoflavones by themselves, rather than isoflavones with ISP, protect against loss of spinal bone.

In 1998, Dr. Albertazzi and his associates reported in the *Journal of Obstetrics and Gynecology* the results of their double-blind, placebo-controlled study of 104 postmenopausal women, who were given 60 grams/day of ISP powder with 76 milligrams of isoflavones, which reduced their hot flashes by 45 percent, at the end of a twelve-week trial. This is in contrast to the 30 percent reduction seen in the placebo group. The difference is statistically significant. We still don't have scientific answers determining what varying amounts of isoflavones when added to a fixed amount of ISP will have on hot flashes. Nor do we know the long-term effects of isoflavones when combined with ISP.

Obviously, many soy issues require further research and clarification. We need well-controlled, prospective clinical trials to confirm past findings. In addition, we need to study long-term soy use, particularly in Western cultures where high amounts of soy are not part of our customary diets. As to what action to take before results are in, I advise suggesting that your patients read all they can about soy and soy isoflavones, discuss available data with you, and then make appropriate decisions based on their individual circumstances and needs.

Sincerely,

NEIL SOLOMON, M.D., PH.D.

Resources

American Soybean Association
540 Maryville Centre Drive
Suite 390
St. Louis, MO 63141

Archer Daniels Midland (ADM)
P.O. Box 1470
Decatur, IL 62525

Soyfoods Center
P.O. Box 234
Lafayette, CA 94549
1-510-283-2991

Indiana Soybean Board (ISB)
info@indianasoybeanboard.com
1-800-735-0195

Ohio Soybean Council
P.O. Box 479
Columbus, OH 43216-0479
1-614-249-2492

Missouri Soybean Merchandising Council
P.O. Box 104778
Jefferson City, MO 65110
1-800-662-3261
1-573-635-3819

Simply Soy
http://soyfoods.com/simplysoy/index.html

The Soy Connection
http://stratsoy.ag.uiuc.edu/~md-qssb/soycon.html/

Soyfoods Association of America
1 Sutter St. Suite 300
San Francisco, CA 94104
1-415-393-9697

United Soybean Board
P.O. Box 419200
St. Louis, MO 63141-9200
1-800-SOY-INFO

United Soybean Board Hotline
1-800-TALK-SOY

Vegging Out
www.execpc.com/~veggie/recipes.html

Vitasoy (USA) Inc.
99 Park Lane
Brisbane, CA 94005
1-800-VITASOY

Glossary of Terms

Alkaline Imbalance: An inequality in the acid/alkaline balance in the body due to diet, lifestyle and environmental habits.

Amino Acids: The building blocks of proteins, eight of which are considered essential—meaning they cannot be made by the human body and must come from dietary sources.

Androgen: Male hormones such as testosterone or androsterone.

Angiogenesis: The generation of new capillaries to feed solid tumors.

Antibodies: Protein molecules produced by B-cells for immune defense; they work by attaching to antigens, such as viruses, and disabling them.

Antioxidant: A substance that prevents damaging oxidation by scavenging for potentially harmful free radicals on a cellular level. Vitamins C and E are antioxidants.

Atherosclerosis: An artery disease resulting from plaque deposits that impede blood flow and may precede a heart attack or stroke.

Autoimmune Disease: A disease that arises because of an immune disorder where antibodies attack one's own healthy tissues and cells.

Bowman-Birk Inhibitor (BBI): A compound found in soy foods that is a protease inhibitor capable of blocking the action of specific enzymes that can promote the growth of tumors.

Carcinogen: Any substance that can stimulate or encourage the growth of cancer.

Cholesterol: A soft, waxy substance produced in the liver or obtained from dietary sources which is essential for the production of sex hormones, cell membranes, and other important body tissues. High levels of circulating cholesterol have been linked to coronary artery disease.

Coronary Artery Disease: The narrowing of arteries that supply the heart with blood due to plaque buildup. If the blockage is severe enough, a heart attack can occur.

Cortisol: A steroidal hormone produced by the adrenal cortex.

Coumestans: A class of phytoestrogenic plants that include bean sprouts, red clover, and sunflower seeds

Daidzein: An isoflavone that has anticancer properties. Daidzein is found in smaller amounts than genistein in the soybean.

Diethylstilbestrol (DES): One of the first synthetic, non-steroidal estrogen drugs and a sad commentary on the hidden dangers of prescription drugs; this chemical increased the risk of vaginal and cervical cancers in women who were exposed to the drug as fetuses.

Diuretic: A medicine or agent used to increase the amount of urine excreted.

Endocrine System: Gladular system of the body that includes the thyroid, adrenal and pituitary glands.

Enzymes: Substances that initiate and control chemical reactions in the body.

Epidemiological Study: A study that looks at the incidence of a disease or condition in a large population and studies possible links with environmental, genetic or dietary factors.

Equol: An estrogenic compound discovered in 1982 that is produced by intestinal bacteria and is similar in structure to human estrogen called estradiol-17. Equol levels are elevated in the urine of people who eat soy foods.

Essential Fatty Acids: Lipid compounds that cannot be made by the body and must be obtained from dietary sources.

Estradiol: The most common circulating hormone in premenopausal women.

Estriol: An estrogenic compound found in the urine of pregnant women; it is made in the placenta and doesn't seem to pose health risks.

Estrogen: A hormone primarily produced in the ovaries that is responsible for female sexual traits and also sustains bone mass, keeps skin soft, controls the menstrual cycle, etc.

Estrogen-Sensitive Tissues: Body tissues that respond to estrogen.

Estrone: The most common circulating hormone in post-menopausal women.

Feedback Cycle: A self-regulatory biological system in which the ouput or response affects the input either positively or negatively, as in the synthesis of some hormones.

Fibrocystic Breasts: Breast tissue showing the development of excess fiberous connective tissue (or fibrosis) associated with dilated glandular structure, as in benign breast cysts.

Folic Acid: A water-soluble vitamin that works closely with vitamin B12 to create healthy red blood cells; it is necessary for the DNA production of all cells in the body and allows the body to use proteins. A deficiency of this vitamin causes anemia and liver problems.

Free Radicals: Unstable molecular structures generated during oxidation in a cell. They are responsible for the cellular damage that results in cancer and other diseases associated with aging.

Genistein: The most abundant soy isoflavone and phytoestrogenic compound, which can act as an estrogen or antiestrogen in the human body. Genistein has a number of therapeutic and disease preventative properties.

Glucoside: Any in a group of glucosides that yields the simple sugar glucose upon hydrolysis.

High-Density Lipoprotein (HDL) Cholesterol: Form of cholesterol beneficial to the body; also known as "good cholesterol."

Hypoglycemia: Abnormally low levels of glucose (simple sugar) in the blood.

Immunologic: Associated with the branch of science dealing with immune response and the immune system.

Indoles: Anticancer compounds found in certain vegetables that can help keep bad estrogen in check.

Ipriflavone: A synthetic isoflavone compound engineered by Japanese scientists and registered as a drug capable of treating bone loss. It is now available as a dietary supplement for osteoporosis prevention and treatment.

Isoflavones: Phytoestrogenic compounds found most abundantly in soy and some other plant foods. Isoflavones have mild estrogenic actions.

Low-Density Lipoprotein (LDL) Cholesterol: Form of cholesterol thought to be detrimental to the body; also known as "bad cholesterol."

Legumes: A food group that includes plants with seed pods such as beans and peas. Soybeans belong to the legume family and contain hundreds of valuable phytonutrients.

Lignin: A binding agent found in plant fibers.

Linoleic Acid: An essential fatty acid that comes from some edible fats and oils and is a component of vitamin F, which is used in vitamins and as an emulsifier.

Linolenic Acid: A polyunsaturated acid made in the body as a metabolite of linoleic acid and commonly used to treat eczema. It is also thought to help prevent heart disease.

Lymphocyte: A type of white blood cell important to the production of antibodies.

Metabolism: Physical and chemical processes in the body through which the body is maintained and energy is created.

Neurotransmitters: Chemicals found in the brain and spinal cord that carry messages between nerve cells.

Oncology: The branch of medicine dealing with tumor origin, growth and treatment.

Osteoporosis: A disease characterized by a loss of bone mass, which results in low bone density and makes bones more susceptible to fractures.

Phenolic Acids: Tannin compounds found in various plant foods, such as carrots, broccoli, cabbage and eggplants, that have antioxidant and anticancer properties.

Phytic Acid: An acid compound occurring naturally in soy and other cereal grains that is used to chelate heavy metals.

Phytochemicals: Biochemicals that come from plants; some of these chemicals are benefical for humans.

Phytoestrogens: Plant compounds capable of exerting a mild estrogenic action in the body.

Precursor: A compound that turns into another active compound through biochemical processes. For examply, beta carotene is considered a precursor compound to vitamin A.

Progesterone: A female hormone that functions in the menstrual cycle to prepare the uterus for a fertilized egg.

Progestin: Any of several steroidal hormones with progesterone-like activity; these include synthetic forms often found in oral contraceptives.

Prolactin: A pituitary hormone that stimulates milk production in mammals.

Protease Inhibitors: Compounds found in some plants like soy that block the action of certain enzymes that promote the growth of tumors.

Protein: Made from amino acids, proteins make up a part of virtually every body cell and regulate the synthesis of hormones and enzymes.

Receptor Site: A protein molecule found on the surface of a cell that recognizes and binds to a specific molecule only.

Serotonin: Neurochemical in the brain that regulates mood, hunger and sleep.

T-Cells: A group of related white blood cells known as lymphocytes that circulate in the blood and regulate immune response to infected or malignant cells.

Testosterone: Male sex hormone that stimulates the growth of male sex organs and sexual traits, as well as sperm.

Transfatty Acids: Artificially formed acids formed when liquid oil is converted to a solid stick. These acids are linked to increased risk for artery disease as well as breast cancer; terms like "hydrogenated" or "partially hydrogenated" found on food labels usually signal the presence of transfatty acids.

Xenoestrogens: A group of synthetic chemicals with estrogenic actions.

Bibliography

Abelow, B.J. et al. "Cross-cultural association between dietary animal protein and hip fracture: a hypothesis." *Calcif Tissue Int.* 50 (1992): 14–18.

Adler, T. "Study reaffirms tamoxifen's dark side." *Sci News.* 4 (June 1994): 356.

Adlercreutz, H. "Phytoestrogens: Epidemiology and a possible role in cancer protection." *Envir Health Persp.* Suppl. 103 (1995): 103–112.

———. "Soybean phytoestrogen intake and cancer risk." *J Nutrition.* 125, no. 3 (1995): 757S–770S.

———. "Diet and breast cancer." *Acta Oncologica.* 31, no. 2 (1992): 175–181.

Adlercreutz, H. and W. Mazur. "Phytoestrogens and western diseases." *Ann of Med.* 29 (1997): 95–120.

Adlercreutz, H. et al. "Dietary phyto-oestrogens and the menopause in Japan." *Lancet.* 339 (1992): 1233.

———. "Lignan and phytoestrogen excretion in Japanese consuming traditional diet." *Scand J Clin Invest.* 48 (1988): 190.

———. "Excretion of the lignans enterolactone and enterodiol and of equol in omnivorous and vegetarian women and in women with breast cancer." *Lancet.* 2 (1982): 1295–1299.

Akiyama, T. et al. "Use and specificity of genistein as inhibitor of protein-kinases." *Meth Enzymol.* 201 (1991): 362–370.

———. "Genistein, a specific inhibitor of tyrosine-specific protein kinase." *J Biol Chem.* 262 (1987): 5592–5595.

Albertazzi, P. et al. "The effect of dietary soy supplementation on hot flashes." *Obstet Gynecol.* 91 (1998): 6–11.

Amaral, M. et al. "Oncostatin-M stimulates tyrosine protein phosphorylation in parallel with the activation of p42MAPK/ERK-2 in Kaposi's cells. Evidence that this pathway is important in Kaposi cell growth." *J Clin Investi.* 92. no. 2 (August 1993): 848–857.

Amer J Epidem. August 15, 1997.

Amer J Epidem. December 1, 1996.

Anderson J. et al. "Genistein and bone: studies in rat models and bone cell lines." Second International Symposium on the Role of Soy in Preventing and Treating Chronic Disease. Brussels, Belgium. Sept 15–18, 1996.

———. "Orally dosed genistein from soy and prevention of cancellous bone loss in two ovariectomized rat models." *J Nutrition.* 125 (1995): 799S.

Anthony, M. et al. "Effects of soy isoflavones on atherosclerosis: potential mechanisms." Bowman Gray School of Medicine of Wake Forest University. Winston-Salem, NC.

Arjmandi, B.H. et al. "Role of soy protein with normal or reduced isoflavone con-

286 / SOY SMART HEALTH

tent in reversing bone loss induced by ovarian hormone deficiency in rats." *Am J Clin Nutr.* Suppl. 68, no. 6 (December 1998): 1358S–1363S.

———. "Dietary soybean protein prevents bone loss in an ovariectomized rat model of osteoporosis." *J Nutrition.* 126 (1996): 161–167.

———. "A soy protein-containing diet prevents bone loss due to ovarian hormone deficiency." Second International Symposium on the Role of Soy in Preventing and Treating Chronic Disease. Brussels, Belgium. Sept 15–18, 1996.

Arnold, S. et al. "Differential interaction of natural and synthetic estrogens with extracellular binding proteins in a yeast estrogen screen steroids." 1997.

———. "Synergistic activation of estrogen receptor with combinations of environmental chemicals." *Science.* 272 (1996): 1489–1492.

Arnot, B. *The Breast Cancer Prevention Diet.* New York: Little Brown and Company, 1998.

Arpel, J. "The female brain hypoestrogenic continuum from the premenstrual syndrome to menopause." *J Reproduct Med.* 41, no. 9 (1996).

Asahi, M. et al. "Thrombin-induced human platelet aggregation is inhibited by protein tyrosine kinase inhibitors." *ST 638 Genist.* 309 (February 1992): 10–14.

Asidy, A. et al. "Biological effects of isoflavones in young women." *Brit J Nutri.* 74, no. 4 (October 1995): 587–601.

Axelson, M. et al. "Soy, a dietary source of the nonsteroidal oestrogen equol in man and animals." *J Endocrin.* 102 (1984): 49–56.

Bagga, D. "Dietary modulation of omega-3.omega-6 polyunsaturated fatty acid ratios in patients with breast cancer." *J Natnl Cancr Insti.* 89, no. 15 (1997): 1123–1131.

Barnes, S. "Rational for the use of genistein containing soy matrices in chemoprevention trails for breast and prostate cancer." *J Cell Biochem.* 22 (1995): 181–187.

———. "Soybeans inhibit mammary tumors in models of breast cancer." *Prog in Clin and Bio Res.* 347 (1990): 239–253.

Barzel, U. "Estrogens in the prevention and treatment of postmenopausal osteoporosis: a review." *Amer J Med.* 85 (1988): 847–850.

Bernstein, L. "Serum hormone levels in premenopausal Chinese women in Shanghai and white women in Los Angeles." *Cancr Cause Contrl.* 1 (1990): 51–58.

Bibbo, et al. "Higher risk of breast cancer in mothers given DES during pregnancy. A twenty-five year follow up study of women exposed to DES during pregnancy." *New Engl J Med.* (298) 1978: 763–767.

"Bioavailability of soybean isoflavones dep ends upon gut microflora in women." *J Nutrition.* 125, no. 9 (1995): 2307–2315.

Blair, H. "Action of genistein and other tyrosine kinase inhibitors in preventing osteoporosis." Second International Symposium on the Role of Soy in Preventing and Treating Chronic Disease. Brussels, Belgium. Sept 15–18, 1996.

Blair, H. et al. "Variable effects of tyrosine kinase inhibitors on avian osteoclastic activity and reduction of bone loss in ovariectomized rats." *J Cell Biochem.* 61 (1996): 629–637.

Boulet, M. et al. "Climacteric and menopause in seven southeast Asian countries." *Maturitis.* 19 (1994): 157–176.

Bowen, R. et al. "Antipromotional effect of the soybean isoflavone genistein." *Proc Am Assoc Cancer Res.* 34 (1993): 555.

Bradlow, H. et al. "Indole-3 carbinol: a novel approach to breast cancer prevention." *Ann New York Acad of Sci.* 1996: 768.

Brandi, M. "Ipriflavone: new insights into its mechanism of action on bone remodeling." *Calcif Tissue Int.* 52 (1993): 151–152.

———. "Flavonoids: biochemical effects and therapeutic applications." *Bone Min.* 19 (1992): S3–S14.

Brann, D. "Progesterone: the forgotten hormone." *Persp Bio Med.* 34, no. 4 (1993): 642.

Breslau, N. et al. "Relationship of animal protein-rich diet to kidney stone formation and calcium metabolism." *J Clin Endocrinol Metab.* 66 (1988): 140–146.

Brown, N. et al. "Prepubertal genistein treatment modulates TGF-alpha, EGF and EGF receptor mRNAs and proteins in the rat mammary gland." *Mol Cell Endcrn.* 144, no. 1 and 2 (1998): 149–165.

Burke, G. "The potential use of a dietary soy supplement as a post-menopausal hormone replacement therapy." Second International Symposium on the Role of Soy in Preventing and Treating Chronic Disease. Brussels, Belgium. Sept 15–18, 1996.

Cai, Q. and H. Wei. "Effect of dietary genistein on antioxidant enzyme activities in SENCAR mice." *Nutri and Cancr.* 25, no. 1 (1996): 1–7.

Calvert, G.D. et al. "A trial of the effects of soya-bean flour and soya-bean saponins on plasma lipids, faecal bile acids and neutral sterols in hypercholesterolaemic men." *Br J Nutr.* 45 (1981): 277–281.

Campagnoli, C. et al. "Progestins and breast cancer risk." *Zentralbl Gynakol.* 119, no. 2 (1997): 38–42.

Caragay, A.B. "Cancer preventive foods and ingredients." 1992, *Food Techn.* 46 (1992): 65–68.

Carlsen, E. et al. "Evidence for decreasing quality of semen during last 50 years." *Brit Med Jrnl.* 305 (1992): 609–613.

Carroll, et al. "Soy consumption and cholesterol reduction: review of animal and human studies." *J Nutrition.* 123, no. 3S (1995): 594–597.

Cassidy, A. et al. "Biological effects of isoflavones in young women." *Brit J of Nutri.* 74, no. 4 (1995): 587–601.

———. "Biological effects of a diet of soy protein rich in isoflavones on the menstrual cycle of premenopausal women." *Am J Clin Nutr.* 60, no. 3 (September 1994): 333–340.

Cauley, J. "Hormone replacement therapy and osteoporosis." Second

International Symposium on the Role of Soy in Preventing and Treating Chronic Disease, Brussels, Belgium, Sept 15–18, 1996.

Cauley, J. et al. "Estrogen replacement therapy and fractures in older women: a prospective study." *Ann Intern Med.* 122 (1995): 9–16.

Cave, W. "Dietary omega-3 polyunsaturated fats and breast cancer." *Nutrition.* 12, no. 1 (1996): S39–S42.

Chapuy, M. et al. "Calcium and vitamin D supplements: effect on calcium metabolism in elderly people." *Am J Clin Nutri.* 6 (1987): 324–328.

Clarkson, T.B. et al. "The potential of soybean phytoestrogens for postmenopausal hormone replacement therapy." *Proc Soc Exp Biol Med.* 217, no. 3 (March 1998): 365–368.

Clayton S. et al. "Insulin-like growth factors control the regulation of estrogen and progesterone receptor expression by estrogens." *Mol and Cell Endocrin.* 128, no. 1 and 2 (1997): 57–68.

Colborn, T. et al. "Developmental effects of endocrine-disrupting chemicals in wildlife and humans." *Environ. Health Perspect.* 101 (1993): 378–384.

Colditz, G. et al. "The use of estrogens and progestins and the risk of breast cancer in postmenopausal women." *N Engl J Med.* 332, no. 24 (June 15 1995): 1589–1593.

Conrad, C. and M. Laux N.D. *Natural Woman Natural Menopause.* Harper Collins, 1997.

Costello, C. and E. Lynn. "Estrogenic substances from plants: Glycyrrhiza." *J Amer Pharm Soc.* 39 (1950): 177–180.

Dalais, F. "Soy and Menopause." *Soy Connection.* 5 (1997): 1 & 4.

Dalais, F. et al. "Dietary soy supplementation increases vaginal cytology maturation index and bone mineral content in postmenopausal women." Second International Symposium on the Role of Soy in Preventing and Treating Chronic Disease. Brussels, Belgium. Sept 15–18, 1996.

Darj, E. et al. "Liver metabolism during treatment with estradiol and natural progesterone." *Gyn End.* 7, no.2 (June 1993): 111.

deCatanzaro, D. and E. Macniven. "Psychogenic pregnancy disruptions in mammals." *Neurosci and Biobehav Revs.* 16, no. 1 (Spring 1992): 43–53.

Duker, E. et al. "Effects of extracts from Cimicifuga racemosa on gonadotropin release in menopausal women and ovariectomized rats." *Planta Medica.* 57, no. 5 (1991): 420–424.

Eden, J. et al. "Effects of diet supplement with wheat bran on serum estrogen levels in the follicular and luteal phases of the menstrual cycle." *Nutrition.* 13 (1997):6.

———. "Hormonal effect of isoflavones." Second International Symposium on the Role of Soy in Preventing and Treating Chronic Disease. Brussels, Belgium. Sept 15–18, 1996.

Endocrinology (USA). 137, No.4 (1996): 1313–1318.

Erdman, J. et al. "Short-term effects soy soybean isoflavones on bone in postmenopausal women." Second International Symposium on the Role of Soy in Preventing and Treating Chronic Disease. Brussels, Belgium. Sept 15–17, 1996.

European workshop on the impact of endocrine disruptors on human health and wildlife. Report EUR 17549. Environment and Climate Research Program of DG XII of the European Commission. 1997.

Setchell, K. et al. "Exposure of infants to phytoestrogens from soy-based infant formula." *Lancet.* 349, no. 9070 (1997): 23–27.

Fanti, O. et al. "Systematic administration of genistein partially prevents bone loss in ovariectomized rats in a non-estrogen-like mechanism." Second International Symposium on the Role of Soy in Preventing and Treating Chronic Disease. Brussels, Belgium. Sept 15–18, 1996.

Felson, D. et al. "The effect of postmenopausal estrogen therapy on bone density in elderly women." *N Eng J Med.* 329 (1993): 1141–1146.

Forsythe, W. "Soy Protein, Thyroid Regulation and Cholesterol Metabolism." *J Nutrition.* 123, no. 3S (1995): 619–623.

Fry, D. "Reproductive effects in birds exposed to pesticides and industrial chemicals." *Environ Health Perspect.* 103 (1995): 165–171.

Fry, D. and K. Toone. "DDT-induced feminization of gull embryos." *Science.* 213 (1981): 922–924.

Gao, Y. and M. Yamaguchi. "Zinc enhancement of genistein's anabolic effect on bone components in elderly female rats." *Gen Pharmac.* 2 (1998): 199–202.

Goblitz, P. "Traditional soy foods: processing and products." *J Nutrition.* 123, no. 3S (1995): 570–572.

Godsand, I. and D. Crook. "Update on metabolic effects of steroidal contraceptives and their relationship to cardiovascular disease risk." *Amer J Obst Gyn.* (170) 1994: 1528–1536.

Goodman, M.T. et al. "Association of soy and fiber consumption with the risk of endometrial cancer." *Am J Epidemiology.* 146, no. 4 (August 15 1997): 294–306.

Graf, E. and J. Eaton. "Antioxidant functions of phytic acid." *Free Rad Biol Med.* 8 (1990): 61–69.

Guillette, L. et al. "Developmental abnormalities of the gonad and abnormal sex hormone concentrations in juvenile alligators from contaminated and control lakes in Florida." *Environ Health Perspect.* 102 (1994): 680-688.

Haenszel, W. et al. "Stomach cancer among Japanese in Hawaii." *JNCI.* 49 (1972): 969–988.

Harding, C. et al. "Dietary soy supplementation is oestrogenic in menopausal women." Second International Symposium on the Role of Soy in Preventing and Treating Chronic Disease. Brussels, Belgium. Sept 15–18, 1996.

Harris, C. et al. "The estrogenic activity of phthalate esters in vitro." *Environ Health Perspect.* 105 (1997): 802–811.

Hawrylewicz, et al. "Soy and experimental cancer: animal studies." *J Nutrition.*

123, no. 3S (1995): 709–712.

Hayakawa, K. et al. "Effects of soybean oligosaccharides on human fecal flora." *Micro Ecol in Health and Disease.* 3 (1990): 293–303.

Heaney, R.P. "Calcium in the prevention and treatment of osteoporosis." *J Int Med.* 231 (1992): 169–180.

Heber, D. et al. "Cholesterol-lowering effects of a proprietary Chinese red-yeast-rice dietary supplement." *Am J Clin Nutr.* 69, no. 2 (February 1999): 231–236.

Henderson, C. W. "Tofu and risk of breast cancer in Asian-Americans." 1999.

Hernandez, A. et al. "Caffeine and other predictors of bone density." *Epidemiology.* 4 (1993): 128.

"Hormone supplements add to cancer risk." *USA Today.* January 25, 2000.

Horowitz, M, et al. "Biochemical effects of calcium supplementation in post-menopausal osteoporosis." *Euro J Clin Nutr.* 42 (1988): 775–778.

Hu J. et al. "Diet and cancer of the colon and rectum: a case-control study in China." *Inter J Epidemiol.* 20 (1991): 362–367.

Hughes, C. "Phytochemical mimicry of reproductive hormones and modulation of herbivore fertility by phytoestrogens." *Environ Health Perspect.* (1988): 171–175.

Hunter, D. "Plasma organochlorine levels and the risk of breast cancer." *N Eng J Med.* (1997): 1253–1258.

Hutchins, Andrea. "Urinary phytoestrogen and lignan excretion after consumption of fermented and unfermented soy products." *J Amer Diet Assoc.* (May 1995): 545–551.

Ingram D. et al. "Case-control study of phyto-oestrogens and breast cancer." *Lancet.* 350, no. 9083 (October 4 1997),: 990–994.

Irvine, C. et al. "The potential adverse effects of soybean phytoestrogens in infant feeding." *NZ Med J.* 108 (1995): 208–209.

Ishihara, M. "Effect of gamma oryzanol on serum lipid peroxide level and climacteric disturbances." *Asi-Oceania Jour Obstet Gynaecol.* 10, no. 3 (1984): 317.

Ito, A. "Is miso diet effective for radiatin injuries?" *MisoSci and Tech.* (39) 1991: 71–84.

Ito, A. et al. "Effects of soy products in reducing risk of spontaneous and neutron-induced liver tumors in mice." *Int J. Oncol.* 2 (1993): 773–776.

Jacobson, J. et al. "Effects of exposure to PCBs and related compounds on growth and activity in children." *Neurotoxicol Teratol.* 12 (1990): 319–326.

———. "Effects of in-utero exposure to polychlorinated biphenyls and related contaminants on cognitive functioning in young children." *J Pediatr.* 116 (1990): 38–45.

Jeng, M.H. et al. "Estrogenic potential of progestins in oral contraceptives to stimulate human breast cancer cell proliferation." *Cancer Res.* 52, no. 23 (December 1 1992): 6539–6546.

Kaaks, R. "Nutrition, hormones and breast cancer: is insulin the missing link?" *Cancr Caus Contr*. 6 (1996): 605–25.

Kalkhoven E. et al. "Synthetic progestins induce breast tumor cell lines." *Molec Cell Endocrin*. 102 (1994): 45.

Karmali, R. "Omega-3 fatty acids and cancer." *J Int Med*. 225, no. 1 (1989): 197–200.

Kelce, W. et al. "Persistent DDT metabolite p,p'-DDE is a potent androgen receptor antagonist." *Nature*. 375 (1995): 581–585.

Kennedy, Ann. "The evidence for soybean products as cancer preventive agents." *J Nutrition*. 123, no. 3S (1995): 733–743.

Koo, L.C. "Dietary habits and lung cancer risk among Chinese females in Hong Kong who never smoked." *Nutr Cancer*. 11 (1988): 155–172.

Kramer, V. et al. "In vitro estrogenicity and anti-estrogenicity of hydroxylated chlorinated biphenyls in human breast tumor (MCF-7) cells." *Organohalogen Compounds*. 20 (1994): 475–480.

Kritchevsky, D. "Dietary protein, cholesterol and atherosclerosis: a review of the early history." *J Nutrition*. 123, no. 3S (1995): 589–593.

Kroon, UB et al. "The effects of transdermal estradiol and oral conjugated estrogens on haemostasis variables." *Thrombosis Haemostasis*. 71, no. 4 (April 1994): 420–423.

Lancet. 350, no. 9083 (October 4 1997): 990–994.

Lange C. et al. "Hypothesis: progesterone primes breast cancer cells for cross-talk with proliferative or antiproliferative signals." *Mol Endocrinol*. 13, no. 6 (June 13 1999): 829–836.

Lauritzen, C. et al. "Treatment of premenstrual tension syndrome with Vitex agnus castus. Controlled, double-blind study versus pyridoxine." *Phytomedicine*. 4, no. 3 (1997): 183–189.

Lee, J. R. *Natural Progesterone: The Multiple Roles of a Remarkable Hormone*. Revised. California: BLL Publishing, 1993.

———. *What Doctors May Not Tell You About Menopause*. New York: Warner Books, 1996.

Licata A. "Prevention and osteoporosis management." *Cleveland Clin J Med*. 61 (1994): 451–460.

Lock, M. "Contested meaning of the menopause." *Lancet*. 337 (1991): 1270–1272.

Love, Susan. *Dr. Susan Love's Hormone Book*. New York: Random House, 1997.

Lu, L-J. "Effects of one month of soy consumption on circulatory steroids in men." University of Texas Medical Branch.

Marsh, A. et al. "Vegetarian lifestyle and bone mineral density." *Amer J Clin Nutr*. 48 (1988): 837.

Marshall, E. "Search for a killer: focus shifts from fat to hormones." *Science*. 259 (1993): 818–821.

Messina, M. et al. *The Simple Soybean and Your Health*. New York: Avery

Publishing, 1994.

Messina, M. "Modern applications for an ancient bean: soybeans and the prevention and treatment of chronic disease." *J Nutrition*. 123, no. 3S (1995): 567–569.

———. "The role of soy products in reducing risk of cancer." *JNCI*. 83, no. 8 (1991): 541–46.

Michnovich, Jon and D. S. Klein. *How to Reduce Your Risk of Breast Cancer*. Warner Books, 1996.

Mindell, Earl. *Earl Mindell's Soy Miracle*. Fireside/Simon & Schuster, 1995.

Murkies, A. et al. "Dietary flour supplementation decreases post-menopausal hot flashes: effect of soy and wheat." *Maturitas*. 21 (1995): 189–195.

Nagai, M. et al. "Relationship of diet to the incidence of esophageal and stomach cancer in Japan." *Nutr Cancer*. 3 (1982): 257–268.

Nagel, S. et al. "Relative binding affinity-serum modified access (RBA-SMA) assay predicts the relative in vivo activity of the xenoestrogens bisphenol A and octylphenol." *Environ Health Perspect*. 105, no. 1 (1997): 70–76.

Nananda, F. "Patient specific decisions about hormone replacement therapy in post-menopausal women." *J Amer Med Assoc*. 277, no. 14 (1997), 1997.

Nesbitt, P. and L. Thompson. "Lignans in homemade and commercial products containing flaxseed." *Nutr and Cancr*. 1997, 29(3): 222–227.

Neuberger, et al. "Oestrogenic effects of plant foods in postmenopausal women." *Brit Med J*. (1990): 301.

Nicholas L, et al. "Stimulatory influence of soy protein isolate on breast secretion in pre- and postmenopausal women." Department of Epidemiology and Biostatistics, University of California, San Francisco, California 94142 0560.

Nielsen, F.H. "Boron—an overlooked element of potential nutritional importance." *Nutr Today*. (January/February 1988): 4–7.

Nielson, F. et al. "Effect of dietary boron on mineral, estrogen and testosterone metabolism in postmenopausal women." *Fed Am Soc Exp Biol*. 1, no. 5 (1987): 394–397.

Park, C. "Calcium metabolism." *Jour Amer Coll Nutr*. 8 (1989): 46S–53S.

Persky and V. Horn. "Epidemiology of soy and cancer: perspectives and directions." *J Nutrition*. 123, no. 3S (1995): 709–712.

Peterson, G. and S. Barnes. "Genistein inhibits both estrogen and growth factor-stimulated proliferation of human breast cancer cells." *Cell Growth Different*. 7, no. 10 (1996): 1345–1351.

Petrakis, N. et al. "Stimulatory influence of soy protein isolate on breast secretion in pre- and postmenopausal women." *Cancr Epidem Biomark Prevent*. 5 (1996): 785–794.

Phipps, W. et al. "Effects of flaxseed ingestion on the menstrual cycle." *J Clin Endocrin Metab*. 77 (1993): 1215.

Potter, S. "Overview of proposed mechanism for the Hypocholesterolemic Effects of Soy." *J Nutrition*. 123, no. 3S (1995): 606-611.

————. "Prospective study of estrogen replacement therapy and risk of breast cancer in postmenopausal women." *JAMA.* 264, no. 20 (1990): 2648–2653.

Potter, S. et al. "Soy protein and isoflavones: their effects on blood lipids and bone mineral density in postmenopausal women." *Am J Clin Nutr.* 1998. (in press)

Prince, R. et al. "Prevention of postmenopausal osteoporosis: a comparative study of exercise, calcium supplementation, and hormone-replacement therapy." *N Eng J Med.* 325 (1991): 1189–1195.

Raines, E. and R. Ross. "Biology of atherosclerotic plaque formation: possible role of growth factors in lesion development and potential impact of soy." *J Nutrition.* 123, no. 3S (1995): 624–630.

Rao and Sung. "Saponins as Anticarcinogens." *J Nutrition.* 123, no. 3S (1995): 717–723.

Riggs, B. "A new option for treating osteoporosis." *N Eng J Med.* 323 (1990): 124–125.

Roberts, P. "The menopause and hormone replacement therapy: views of women in general practice receiving hormone replacement therapy." *Brit J Gen Pract.* 41, no. 351 (October 1991): 421–424.

Rose, D. P. "Dietary fiber, phytoestrogens and breast cancer." *Nutrition.* 8, no. 1 (1992): 47–51.

Rose, D. P., et al. "High fiber diet reduces serum estrogen concentrations in premenopausal women." *Amer J Clin Nutr.* 54, no. 3 (1991): 520–525.

Rossignol, A. and H Bonnlander. "Prevalence and severity of the premenstrual syndrome. Effects of foods and beverages that are sweet or high in sugar content." *J Reprod Med.* 3 (February 1991): 131–136.

Safe, S. "Environmental and dietary estrogens and human health: is there a problem." *Environ Health Perspect.* 103 (1995): 346–351.

Schairer, C. et al. "Menopausal estrogen and estrogen-progestin replacement therapy and breast cancer risk." *JAMA.* 283, no. 4 (January 26 2000).

Sellman, S. *Hormone Heresy: What Women MUST Know About Their Hormones.* Get Well International, 1997.

Shekhar, P. "Environmental estrogen stimulation of growth and estrogen receptor function in preneoplastic and cancerous human breast cell lines." *J Nat Canc Inst.* 89, no. 23 (1997): 1997.

Shen F. et al. "Tamoxifen and genistein synergistically down-regulate signal transduction and proliferation in estrogen receptor-negative human breast carcinoma MDA-MB-435 cells." *Anticancr Res.* 19, no. 3A (May-June 1999): 1657–1662.

Sher, A. and A. Rahman. "Role of diet on the enterohepatic recycling of estrogen in women taking contraceptive pills." *J Pakistan Med Assoc.* 44, no. 9 (1994): 213–215.

Shir, Y. et al. "Neuropathic pain following partial nerve injury in rats is suppressed by dietary soy." *Neurosci Lett.* 9240, no. 2 (January 1998): 73–76.

Singh, R.B. et al. "Hypolipidemic and antioxidant effects of Commiphora mukul (gugulipid) as an adjunct to dietary therapy in patients with hypercholesterolemia." *Cardiovasc Drugs Ther*. 8, no. 4 (August 1994): 659–664.

Sirtori et al. "Soy and cholesterol reduction: clinical experience." *J Nutrition*. 123, no. 3S (1995): 598–605.

Steele et al. "Cancer chemoprevention agent development strategies for genistein." *J Nutrition*. 123, no. 3S (1995): 713–716.

Steinberg, S. et al. "Tryptophan in the treatment of late luteal phase dysphoric disorder: a pilot study." *J Psych and Neurosci*. 19, no. 2 (March 1994): 114–119.

———. "Studies spark tamoxifen controversy." *Sci News*. 26 (February 1994): 133.

Stoll, B. "Eating to beat breast cancer: potential role for soy supplements." *Ann of Oncol*. 8 (1997): 223–225.

Survey Commissioned by MotherNature.com and released for Women's Health Care Month.

Swanson, C.A. et al. "Dietary determinants of lung-cancer risk: results from a case-control study in Yunnan province, China." *Int J. Cancer*. 50 (1992): 876–880.

Thomson, J. et al. "Relationship between nocturnal plasma estrogen concentration and free plasma tryptophan in perimenopausal women." *Jour Endocrinol*. 3 (1977): 395–396.

Thune, M. et al. *N Eng J Med*. (May 1 1997).

Toppari, J. et al. "Male reproductive health and environmental xenoestrogens." *Environ Health Perspect*. Suppl. 104, no. 4 (1996): 741–803.

United States Environmental Protection Agency. "Special report on environmental endocrine disruption: an effects assessment and analysis." *EPA*. 630/R-96/012 (1997): 1–111.

United States Senate Document 264, Mineral Depletion in Soils, second session of the 74th Congress (1936).

US 1997 Soyfoods Directory Indiana Soybean Development Council.

Verma, S. "Curcumin and genistein, plant natural products show synergistic inhibitory effects on the growth of human breast cancer MCF-7 cells induced by estrogenic pesticides." *Biochem and Biophys Commun*. 233 (1997): 692–696.

Wakai, K. et al. "Dietary intake and sources of isoflavones among Japanese [In Process Citation] Department of Preventive Medicine, Nagoya University School of Medicine." *Nutr Cancr*. 33, no. 2 (1999): 139–145.

Watanabe, Y. et al. "A case-control study of cancer of the rectum and the colon." *Nippon Shokakibyo Gakkai Zasshi*. 81 (1984): 185–193.

Wei, H. "Antioxidant and anti-promotional effects of the soybean isoflavone genistein." *Proceed Society Exper Bio Med*. 208 (1995): 124.

Widhalm, K. "Hypocholesterolemic effects of soy in children." Dept. of Pediatrics, University of Vienna, Austria.

Wilcox and Blumenthal. "Thrombotic mechanisms in atherosclerosis: potential impact of soy proteins." *J Nutrition.* 123, no. 3S (1995): 631–638.

Wilcox, G. et al. "Estrogenic effects of plant foods in postmenopausal women." *Brit Med J.* 301 (1990): 905–906.

Witschi, H. et al. "Modulation of lung tumor development in mice with the soybean-derived Bowman-Birk protease inhibitor." *Carcinogenesis.* 10 (1989): 2275–2277.

Witte, J. et al. "Diet and premenopausal bilateral breast cancer: a case-control study." *Breast Cancr Res Treat.* 42 (1997): 243–251.

Wolff, M. and P. Toniolo. "Environmental organochlorine exposure as a potential etiologic factor in breast cancer." *Environ Health Perspect.* 103, no. 7 (1995): 141–145.

Woods, M. et al. "Effect of a dietary soy bar on menopausal symptoms." Second International Symposium on the Role of Soy in Preventing and Treating Chronic Disease. Brussels, Belgium, Sept 15–18, 1996.

Wu, A. H. et al. Department of Preventive Medicine, University of Southern California, Los Angeles, California.

Wurtman, R. and J. "Carbohydrates and depression." *Sci Amer.* (January 1989): 68–75.

Xu, X. "Bioavailability of soybean isoflavones depends upon gut microflora in women." *J Nutrition.* 125, no. 9 (1995): 2307–2317.

Yingman, Y. et al. "A study of the etiological factors in gastric cancer in Fuzhou City." *Chinese J Epidemiol.* 7 (1986): 48–50.

You W. C. et al. "Diet and high risk of stomach cancer in Shandong, China." *Cancer Res.* 48 (1988): 3518–3523.

Zava, D. "Estrogenic and anti-proliferative properties of genistein and other flavonoids in human breast cancer cells in vitro." *Nutr and Cancr.* 27, no. 1 (1997): 31–40.

Zeigler, Regina. "Quantifying estrogen metabolism." *Environ Health Perspect.* 105, no. 3 (1997).

Zhy, D. "Dong quai." *Amer Jour Clin Med.* 15, no. 3–4 (1987): 1987.

Index